blood Whispers

L.A.

WRITERS

ON

AIDS

EDITED BY

TERRY

WOLVERTON

books

Silverton
Books
and
The Gay
and
Lesbian
Community
Services
Center

THE CENTER

Los Angeles
1991

Grateful acknowledgement is made to the authors for permission to reprint previously published material:

"At Risk" by Gil Cuadros, was previously published in *Asklepios.*

"RM#" by Gil Cuadros, was previously published in *Art X Press,* Vol. 1, No. 1, 1990.

"Wild Ride" by Bia Lowe, was previously published in *The Western Humanities Review,* Vol. XLIV, No. 3, 1990.

"Ed Dying" and "40" by Paul Monette, were previously published in *Poets for Life* (Crown Publishing Group, 1989).

"Caring Without Answers" by Robin Podolsky, was previously published in *Caregiver: A Publication of the AIDS Healthcare Foundation,* Vol. 1, No. 5, 1990.

"Obituary – Chris Brownlie" by Doug Sadownick, was previously published in *L.A. Weekly,* Vol. 12 No. 1, December 8–14, 1989.

~

TERRY WOLVERTON WISHES TO EXPRESS GRATITUDE TO THE FOLLOWING INDIVIDUALS FOR THEIR ASSISTANCE IN REALIZING THIS PROJECT: JULIE ANDERSON, NANCY ANGELO, LAUREN JARDINE, CHERYL MENDOZA, TORIE OSBORN, AND JULIA SALAZAR. THIS PUBLICATION IS MADE POSSIBLE IN PART BY GRANTS FROM THE CITY OF LOS ANGELES CULTURAL AFFAIRS DEPARTMENT; THE CALIFORNIA ARTS COUNCIL, A STATE AGENCY; AND THE NATIONAL ENDOWMENT FOR THE ARTS, A FEDERAL AGENCY; AND THROUGH THE SUPPORT OF THE GAY AND LESBIAN COMMUNITY SERVICES CENTER.

Cover and Book Design
S *o* S : SUSAN SILTON, Los Angeles

Printed in an edition of 1000 copies
Typeset on Macintosh IIx in Adobe Garamond
Linotronic Output by Electric Pencil, Los Angeles

Printed in the United States of America
Library of Congress Catalog Card Number: 91-090365

ISBN 0-9629528-0-X

Table of Contents

PART TWO: TESTIMONIES

PART THREE: TALES

Foreword

The Center is very proud to initiate this anthology as a means of helping writers and poets to share their vision with the public at large and with others whose lives are forever changed by the presence of HIV and AIDS.

We have been fortunate to feature the extraordinary talents of artist-in-residence Terry Wolverton in an innovative writing project focusing on issues of HIV in the gay and lesbian community. Terry's work has helped to develop meaningful and gifted literary responses to the human drama of AIDS in our community. Since October 1988, the artist-in-residence program has enjoyed the support of the California Arts Council, the National Endowment for the Arts, and the Center's Education Department.

The Gay and Lesbian Community Services Center ("The Center") was founded in 1971, soon after the national groundswell of pride and politics begun by Stonewall became a part of our lives. Los Angeles is richly honored to be the home of the oldest and largest center of its kind in the world, sensitive to the co-sexual and multi-cultural environment of the diverse gay and lesbian communities. The Center has always been on the cutting edge of HIV services, and serves more HIV-affected people than any other HIV service provider in Los Angeles County. Programs range the continuum from prevention to treatment, including: *STOP AIDS Los Angeles, West Hollywood CARES, Computerized aids Information Network (CAIN), West Hollywood HIV Healthcare Center, Addiction Recovery Services for HIV-affected, Youth Services, Legal Services, Bi-lingual AIDS information/referral services, HIV Anonymous Testing, Philip Mandelker AIDS Prevention Clinic,* and the *ACCESS Program (Counseling Department.)*

~ FOREWARD ~

The Center is a vibrant, central organizing hub for the Los Angeles community, and is deeply committed to the arts and their meaning in our lives. This anthology, for which we received support from the City of Los Angeles Cultural Affairs Department, represents the best and brightest of L.A.'s established and emerging writers, and we are delighted to share it with you.

TORIE OSBORN

EXECUTIVE DIRECTOR

GAY AND LESBIAN COMMUNITY SERVICES CENTER

Introduction

for David Moores,
and for all my writing students
who struggle with HIV

I could do nothing but watch as his face grew grey, as his slender frame was whittled like a scrap of balsa, as the grape blotch spread over his face like a stain. Nothing but watch and try to feed his fragile hope, a hope which could not succor me.

I met him on the very first night of my writing workshop, a workshop for people with HIV. I began this class because I'd grown uncomfortable with the insularity I felt as a lesbian in this time of AIDS. I wanted to tear the web of separation, I wanted to do something. He was charming, gregarious, astute, and as the weeks progressed I learned that he had a talent for fiction, the ability to fashion complex characters and move them through the world.

In the first year, all went well for him. What began as a class exercise mushroomed into more than a hundred pages, and he began to entertain seriously my suggestion that he might be writing a novel. A novel about a man with AIDS. I could see the book in my mind; I wanted to finger its pages, feel the weight of its spine in my hands. I had to temper my impulse to push him too hard, too fast; I felt a sense of urgency, of limited time, but as a teacher I know good writing is like bread dough: it must have time to rise and swell, to be worked over and over, kneaded and turned, and time to rise again. It can't be rushed.

Partway into the second year, he missed several weeks of class. When he returned he was thinner, had been in the hospital, he explained. He continued to work on the novel, always eager to read aloud in class; his stack of pages doubled. A few months later, another hospitalization, from which he emerged still weaker, with ash blotting his tanned complexion. Not long after that he reported in class that his T-cell count was 8. Then he stopped coming to the weekly sessions, although he did summon the strength to join the group for a reading over the summer.

We kept in touch by phone. His health rose and fell in waves, cresting ever lower after each descent. He still sometimes talked about the book, but he was just too tired, he said, to do much more than think about it. Perhaps he lost faith in words, in their power to save him; perhaps he could not imagine an ending that did not include his own.

His, of course, is just one story. One more voice silenced, one more book unpenned. There are too goddamned many of these stories.

As a writer, a teacher, an editor, there is little I can do, but what little I can I must do: Keep faith in the power of words, while accepting their terrible limits. Keep on feeding hope, even as the hopeful are devoured. Keep alive the stories of those whose voices have been drowned by the treacherous whispers in the blood.

TERRY WOLVERTON

EDITOR

PART ONE

Tributes

Ed Dying

by Paul Monette

Hate is an old man fucking, arduous
and half a bone, but I work at it
like Sophie Tucker, a last geriatric fling
like pushing a car uphill with a rope.
Hate the Reagans and their facile cancers,
all straight people with lives and my brothers
who flee to the continent having buried
their allotment. This is the rage of the 8th
year, bent out of shape, crazily displaced,
yelling at the queerest people because
the scum politicos of the NIH are out
of reach, funding the end of the world.
I massacre whoever gets in my small way – check
lost in the mail, promise of shirts Friday,
876-4466 my Thrifty druggist rings busy busy
and I need refills like a one-arm bandit,
that kind of thing. As for Ed, Ed is dying
by phone, dwindling in secret, doing without
spunk and visitors. I leave word weekly
on his machine, reports of my latest tantrum,
a recent self-immolation in the Mayfair checkout.
For months there is no reply, but we are
light-years beyond good manners, Ed and I,
loathing bullshit so and the comfort of sunny
disposition. Checked in the day Rita Hayworth died:
Hi Ed, poor Gilda, huh? My only friend who knows
how blonde the lady from Shanghai was and why
it matters so. Publicity errs on the bright side
always, burning for us to have a good time.

Ed who has met them all – Cary, Hitch, Her Serene
Highness – is the last living link between us
poor queens and To *Catch a Thief,* speaking of Eden
lost. Now we are all on the last train out,
fleeing fleeing, diamonds up our ass, the past
curling like smoke as Marlene drags her last
Gitane. Even as Ed is dying, in Washington
everyone eats his boogers and Mormons file
the plague under Pest Control, Reagan's colon
clear as a bagpipe, his sausage tumors
replicated in lifelike vinyl for souvenirs.
Then suddenly over New Year's Eve: *This is Ed.*
Thank you for all your messages. I love
your rage. So I hate mostly for Ed's sake now,
and the old man fucking with his dick in a brace
has mounted a bimbo who can't feel it, does it
for fifty, next year will do it for thirty-five
and eat his shorts for an encore. There are easier
ways than all this slamming about, I admit,
but the time comes – say after the third pneumonia,
and they send you home to recuperate with
the wrong dose, 200 fucking milligrams less
than what will make you live again, and ten
days later you're back in stir, starting it all
over, over and over – the time will come
when you prove you are still alive just feeling
anything at all. So sometimes we are wronged
as Lana Turner in the fifties, jilted and stomped,
herded like misfits, the vanishing years aching
like a torrent of smoke thrown by a moonlit train
bound for the chaos of Shanghai. And if we wail
and spew bile we say we are not collaborators,
for Ed would not be dying please without

the complicity of niceness, so many smiling
colon exams. Yes, it's hard to keep it up,
me and this numb member of mine, rutting
while Rome burns, but to hate everything
half-true – including me, especially me –
a nasty temper works like a Spanish fly.
Be hard and cry foul, I order my bad thing,
for we are in enemy hands, buying time like
fallen women in countries torn by the death
grip of keeping things polite. Hate for the same
reason a man might sit and weep: missing Ed.

Excerpt from "downtown," a solo performance work

by Luis Alfaro

Smiley:

I think it's because I'm crazy.
I think it's because I'm Catholic.
I think it's because of buildings.
I think it's because I smile too much.
I think that's why I got picked.

I'm not saying I ain't guilty.
I did it.
I took big steps instead of baby steps and didn't even say mother may I.
I ran the yellow when I should have stopped for the red.
I kept walking past the danger signal ahead.
I was a mean mother fucker when I could have been nice. *(shrugs)*
But I don't think it's my fault.

I blame it on the buildings.
If there weren't so Goddamn many in the city maybe I could have found my way out.
Used to be I knew every building in the city. Now I get off the bus and I'm standing in front of this building that just came out of nowhere.

There are people in this city who run at the sight of a helicopter light. Afraid, I guess, that their sins will show through like the partition at confession. I've never understood it. I run into them. Waving wildly at the sky, "Hey you guys it's me. Waz up?" Then a cop car pinpoints me to a corner and it's all over.

I am so afraid of getting lost in this city.
Another face in a shuffle of millions.
Begging for attention on help lines that ring busy.
Shelters with take-a-number machines.
Social workers that cancel appointments to go to an audition.

I did it for love.
For a mean chingona from Lincoln Heights that I met between two buildings in downtown. When we rode, we went straight to heaven. Like a Led Zepplin song.

Used to live in the dressing room a of swimming school on Hollywood and Western. Used to have to wait until dark to go home. And one day we walked to the corner, bought a little shit, went to Ralph's, swiped some Kraft's macaroni and cheese, went home and shot up.

I always had it in me.
Came out kicking and screaming from the start.

I am a frustrated fifth grader.
I'll give you an example. Two men walk up to my door and both say they're my dad. I look at both of them and say "yeah? prove it."

The first one comes up to me, hugs me, holds me and kisses me on the cheek. I look up at him and say, "Man, you are a sorry assed liar."

The second one comes up to me, slaps me hard on the face, punches me in the stomach, grabs me by the hair and I look up at him and say, "Hi dad."

The first one is heroin.

After that it gets easy.
Because being a good addict is like having a bank account. You buy two hits. One is checking and the other is savings. When you get desperate you dip into the savings a bit.

Me, I never get desperate. You know why? Cause I ain't greedy. I could buy some shit on 5th and Spring, give it away, and still get a hit on 7th and Main. I'm one of the lucky ones. There are about ten lucky people in this city. Me, the Mayor, the lady that runs the car insurance and the man that owns McDonalds. A few others.

I think that's how I got it. Being too generous. But that's okay cause, like, look at Jesus. He was giving away the good shit like crazy and he got the ultimate back stab in history.

But you know what? Sometimes I think it's religion that did it. Like this idea that we all gotta suffer. Standing in this line at County General waiting for my treatment reminds me of my olden days when I was a wild wild one standing in the same line waiting for stitches after a house party that got out of hand. Almost like some angel said, "Sorry fucker, but in God's book the lion lays down with the lamb."

I have this vision of Christ on the cross that I grew up with. But it just ain't real. When I got sick, I had these dreams that Jesus climbs down from that cross and he's wearing khaki's, a pendelton and a bandanna. And he starts walking amongst us. And he comes right up to me and his hand pierces my heart.

And it's funny that just when I really begin to see,
I start losing my eyesight.

AIDS is a funny word. Like someone is really gonna give a shit.
But hey. No regrets rights?

Getting high makes me smile. I forget things easily.
Street corner homeboys walk by and salute me.
Veteranos sigh and wish for the old days of simple Thunderbird highs.
Mexican mothers cackle like chickens at a clothesline.
The future is nothing but the name of a brand new Japanese sports car.
Murals look brand new again.
MacArthur Park is clean.
So are my veins and so is my blood.

And when I'm high I just gotta smile, cause two angels with the faces of social workers lift me up, stick tubes in my veins and they purify my blood. And this blood runs through the City of Angels and makes it all clean again.

And sometimes this city looks like a Las Vegas whore at three o'clock in the morning.
But tonight this city is downtown.
Tonight this city is buildings.
Tonight this city is all lights and nobody gets lost.
Tonight something is going down on every corner.

Tonight the grey suits on Figueroa are running into the big clubs.
Tonight the bus is on time.

Tonight I'm running through these streets. Through Echo Park Lake. Through the Evergreen cemetery down by Lorena. Down on the south side of L.A. by the race track. Down through Chinatown up to Elysian park to look for La Llorona. Down through the streets of El Sereno with the cold cholo gaze staring down a homeboy in enemy territory. Down Pico and the Salvadorian bakeries. Straight into downtown and into the arms of Our Lady. And her arms are big buildings that reach down and hug you.
Oh these memories...

Really, you know what? I blame it on the buildings.

Wild Ride

by Bia Lowe

We were both drop-outs, both floundered in our first year of college and ended up affluent and directionless back in the Bay Area the year after the "Summer of Love." He would stop by my pad around two, after seeing his therapist. With his long greasy hair, long wrinkled raincoat, hollow eyes and high-tops, he was every bit the image of Ichabod Crane-meets-William Burroughs. I was, in my overalls, work shirt, long hair and fringe jacket, the very image of Emma Goldman-meets-Annie Oakley. We'd walk around the city and smoke joints, talking about the corruption in all things Amerikan. The subtext in our conversations was a rebellion against sex roles – a sentiment that was finding its legs with flower power and would soon find its voice with the sexual movements of the seventies. We were struggling to be n*ot* well-adjusted, to discover the selves beneath our years of cotillions, prep schools and proper manners. We elevated childhood as the purer form – a realm where the noble savage romped, unfettered by the likes of Hugh Hefner and Carol Doda. We were resisting assimilation, holding fast to our polymorphous perversity, reclaiming arrested development.

He collected children's books, I collected toys. We were brother and sister in a family for which we hadn't a name.

~

But this is not another homosexual story. I was intending to write about Clark because, even though it's been two years, I'm trying to construct the meaning of his death. The way one constructs the meaning of a dream, by lowering a net and bringing its life writhing to the surface.

~

And dreams often concern death, or the threat of it. The colossal fist of the ocean looms above me, or I'm unable to stop my speeding car though my foot presses, presses the brake. Shrinks would tell me, and have, that these are symbolic representations of feeling states – they don't necessarily mean I'm afraid of the ocean or that I'll die in a car accident.

But sometimes I wonder: out of the many dreams I have, couldn't *one* be prescient? Isn't it possible for some dreams to depict not mere representations, but literal truths? And if so, which dream should I pay attention to? Will there be a time when I'm unable to stop my car and the useless flooring of the brake will seem nightmarishly familiar?

~

There is a ride at Disneyland, a mad ride in an old jalopy, where every wrench in the road is a kind of ticklish jeopardy. And as you career past each hazard, each more hair-raising than the last, you wonder where will it end? When will the hilarity turn to dead-pan adrenaline? Cops pop up from nowhere blowing whistles. Brick walls wobble precariously, and as you rush seemingly headlong into them, they unhinge. You even blast into a courtroom, barely missing the lawyer who swears by heaven he'll sentence you for speeding. But finally you swing screeching into a tunnel, and you realize, perhaps because it's so dark, that this part of the ride is different. Up ahead, the approaching sound of a locomotive and the headlight of its engine bring on the ice of alarm. Surely your car will swerve before you collide. You never suspect that your car will keep going, that the collision will be quiet, painless, that you will keep speeding through the dark.

~

I try to imagine what it means to be dead. As a child I used to believe that when you died, your mind lived on as though nothing had happened. That if, say, you died in a car accident, your immortal mind would imagine you unharmed in the wreckage, that you would continue your business, finish the grocery shopping, return to the ones who love you. Sometimes still I wonder if this might not be true. How could the Ego with all its dazzle and demands simply go poof in the night? A whole luminous life like a dove into a top hat?

And sometimes, especially when I'm driving, I wonder if I might already be dead, if my body has already been struck down, and my experience of driving is really propelled by imagination alone. Undying imagination, like a movie in a dark theater.

~

I watched my cat Lucy die, my companion of fifteen years. Lucy and I kissed each other on the lips and then the vet gave her the drugs. She was out but not yet dead, he said, she had a few minutes left. So I whispered things in her ear, the kinds of things people talk about these days – move toward the light, let this life go, become one with the universe. Her eyes were so dilated they seemed, like the universe, to contain a kind of impending indifference, a hard-edged void that tunneled its way, like the ride at Disneyland, into a continual dark. Then I noticed the cornea of her eyes change from something wet and glassy to something dryer, stippled, already transforming. She was gone. Her body sagged like a puppet with no hand inside it – whatever held all her many cells together was devolving.

All the night before I kept her company, watched her struggle with her pain. And though I wouldn't allow her to, she wanted to go outside, to die as cats know how, alone.

Being human, I couldn't bear it. Dying alone is unthinkable – to be like a beetle on one's back, all arms raking the air, desperate for familiar ground. Or perhaps it's unthinkable because dying *is* being alone, mourning the illusory companionship of one's private glory. The full blaze of a life cools and condenses into simple carbons, the beetle succumbs finally to the inglorious appetites of soil. And there's a distinct lack of applause.

~

I have a photograph of my father and me the year before he died, the year before the Summer of Love. I'm sixteen and he's fifty-three, though he looks at least seventy. He is drinking himself to death. Of course I have the advantage of hindsight, and everything about his appearance is a warning flare to me now, a quarter of a century later. I see he is trying to step out of the picture, away from me and his wife clicking the shutter. He is moving, like the cat, toward a picture in which there is nothing but isolation. I also am trying to escape the picture because his isolation dominates it, and because a part of me has already felt his death, like dreams I laugh off though I keep glancing over my shoulder. I am moving away from him because I am young, and I won't look at what I know.

~

But back to Clark. The fact of the matter is, Clark and I weren't even close. After those few years in San Francisco I moved away to go to school in another city, and ultimately to find my tribe among lesbians. He grew muscles and followed the Dionysian path. Where the sixties had joined us as siblings, the seventies segregated us into distinct species, ghettoized by our sexualities.

Occasionally we'd get together but I found him petty. An hysteric. I think he probably felt my politics had made me twisted and humorless. If you had asked me in the seventies how Clark would die, I probably would have sneered, "Too much sex." Then, I would have thought that a lifestyle like a ride in a wild jalopy could come to no good. But now I question that kind of judgment. Now I question a world spun by moral causality. Now I wonder if, say, the rails on that ride were cracked, if Chaos stood behind the curtain slamming levers, cranking gears, would it matter how slowly, how safely you tried to drive? If, say, something was senseless and awry with the mechanism, if the brick wall refused to unhinge and AIDS was something you got in the pursuit of love, what good is a brake?

The point, if indeed there is one, is this: Life makes us scream with apprehension and delight; if it doesn't, perhaps the ride we're on isn't steep enough. And while part of the body prepares for death, while part of the body is wise to the figure behind the curtain, pulling fractals, cranking the unforeseen, our throats are hoarse with wild laughter and our eyes stream in the thrill of it.

~

Clark's life toward the end was very full. I'd get evidence of its richness in the mail – stories he'd written for the People With AIDS Newsletter, a Christmas card he'd made. I'm looking at that card right now, an exuberant display of arrested development. On the front: a color photograph of Clark and his infant niece dressed up like dinosaurs, surrounded by dinosaur stuffed animals. Inside it reads: "Joyous Eleanorasaurus and Klarkus Crayolatops love you."

He worked at having a family, at rebuilding the very thing that had sent him into therapy two decades earlier. And here he is, a dying man with a baby, dressed like an extinct creature, having the time of his life.

I was told he had his family with him. They listened to his labored breathing, whispered into his ear about letting go, stared into a dark eye already turned inward in search of light. They watched as his story fizzled into the ether like the snowdrifts of television.

~

A few months later I received a packet of wild flower seeds in the mail. This is the second year that Clark's wild flowers are coming up. I mixed the seeds with sand to help them scatter in my garden. It's the same dirt I buried Lucy in. The same dirt that holds the bones of two other cats before her. The dirt of decomposed things – rock, bark, beetles, cats, dinosaurs.

~

There's one last thing about the ride at Disneyland. It doesn't end with the dark tunnel. There's more. A blast of hot air, and the dark cracks open into a riotous bacchanal of demons, hot-pink devils with midriff bulges who bob on walls of lava. They are having, as it were, the time of their lives. A great time, devilishly good. A happy ending to a ride that had been altogether too abbreviated.

I'd like to think that life is resolved in such a place. Not the ethereal retirement home to which all earthly pleasures have been sacrificed, nor the pit of damnation in which the fundamentalists envision the likes of Clark forever wheeling on a rotisserie. I like to think of a livelier place, a place that has no regard for you or me or the Bible – a place in the earth, a seething bacchanal of jocular mildews, horny pollens, ribald bacteria, an arena suitable for the most high-minded of noble savages, full of elemental stuff – seeds, bones, mold.

~

For the last few winters Disneyland has been hosting a fundraiser for the

AIDS Project in L.A. Once a year thousands of homosexuals drive to Anaheim for "Gay Night." If there ever was a more raucous show of arrested development, I've never heard of it. Shrieks and gales of laughter echo through the fog of the Magic Kingdom.

~

After leaving Mr. Toad's Wild Ride, my friend Brian and I head for the Haunted Mansion. There is a long line in front of us that snakes its way through the cemetery. And as we stand in the stream of leather jackets and giggle at the names on the tombstones – "D. Ceest," "Diane Gontahevon." etc. – Brian tells me this joke:

A little boy runs to his mother and asks, "Mommy, is it true that when we are born we come from dust?"

The mother answers, yes.

"And Mommy, is it true that when we die we go back to dust?"

The mother says, yes, that's right. From dust to dust.

"Well, Mommy, come upstairs and look under my bed 'cause someone's either coming or going."

RM#

by Gil Cuadros

John was constantly moved
and each time I returned,
I had to find the station,
to find the room,
the hallways were endless.
Friends cried and strangled the corridors.
I ignored their opened arms,
it made me mad when they held me back
so I'd push them away,
tell them, "He looks great.
You should have seen him yesterday."
They'd wipe their faces unbelieving,
their fingers wrenched the flowers.
I felt like they should die instead,
not John, cornered to the wall, unconscious,
a halo of bare fluorescence.
I explained all the injections and wires
because I needed a distraction
from John's sunken face,
his bones that poked through skin,
his mind taken over by a fungus,
his lips bloody with dehydration,
the tongue cracked and smeared
and a plastic tube shoved down his throat
taped to his mouth
and he was choking,
his veins collapsing,
his brain boiling,
his lungs filling with fluids

and the chemicals made him hallucinate
but they killed.
He slipped in and out,
his hands fluttered, blessing the air.
I held down his arms,
strapped them to the metal rails
as if that would give me peace,
the one thing I prayed.
But all he could do was pick at my palm
pull at the false skin of latex,
stare past me like an animal who avoids the eyes.
Still I tried to whisper sweet thoughts into his ear,
"Baby, I'm at your side, I love you so much,
I don't know what I'll do."
The nurses scattered the onlookers
till I was alone, suffocating.
I was told all I could do was go home and wait,
so I slept in our bed,
pulled his pillow to my face,
dreamt of when our bodies were covered
by the same white sheet.
By the next morning he was gone
and I spent what seemed like a day
chasing him down, out of breath,
his room unlisted, his name erased.

Obituary: Chris Brownlie 1950-1989

by Doug Sadownick

It's hard to lose friends, but it's harder to lose the source of one's inspiration. I got close to Chris Brownlie when I began researching the history of AIDS for an *L.A. Weekly* story almost two years ago. He would call me mornings to take me on an AIDS crash course: "Wake up, girlfriend. It's chemotherapy day at County and we're taking a tour of the dungeons, so don't eat breakfast." We sang at Rev. Carl Bean's black gay and lesbian church. We sat at County AIDS Commission meetings. Always, I felt in the presence of someone who was achieving greatness.

During a recent walk on Venice beach, we checked out the boys while intellectualizing over genocide. He wanted to see gays and lesbians as "teachers" who in their adversity could force Americans to stop repressing their empathy. While Chris thrived on serving his people, he never whitewashed their foibles: emancipation meant a gay psyche that wasn't cloven along color and class lines. He worked at Minority AIDS Project and set up "Blacks Living With AIDS and HIV Disease" with his lover and fellow activist Phill Wilson; he helped to form the AIDS Hospice Foundation with Michael Weinstein to give the poorest a dignified place to die. Having little patience with elitists, even less for the passive, he still got weepy in the hospital recently when recalling how gays had approached him at the West Hollywood Street Fair, thanking him for being heroic. "I love my brothers," he said, "because no one else does, including themselves."

Chris suffered. ("I'm getting creative at this," he muttered last month during seizures.) His creativity escalated as his time diminished, giving his role as "crusader" contradictory dimensions. Through demonstrations, he could humiliate Supervisor Mike Antonovitch into supporting hospice care; the first county-sponsored hospice is named after him, and it is a paragon of institutions. But he could also win the admiration of County/USC honchos, who bowed to community pressure and opened a high-tech AIDS ward. Yet he never made money from his efforts or wore a bureaucratic hat. Most of all, Chris was a thinker; his columns in *The News* make up some of the finest gay political writing in

L.A. Yet he was also, I think, a poet who burned brightly – "AIDS has made me into an artist; every moment feels sublime" – and if you got close, he singed away your own insecurities.

That life force crackled at his deathbed. In spite of the morphine and his failing lungs, he fought a protesting crowd and managed to stand up, kissing Phill. And yet I can find no meaning in his death. Yes, the scene of friends at his bedside – Phill, Michael Weinstein, Albert Ruiz, Mary Adair and Grace Hengst – overpowered me with their love for him. But I ache for my loss, irate that Chris died before an entire society could have benefited from his works. He was a visionary who, had he lived longer, would have fought homophobia, inspired the HIV-infected to be "out," demanding gays and lesbians get off their asses and not let a few do all the work and take all the flak. We lost a leader; they don't just crop up. None of this is an exaggeration. He knew it himself, which is why it disappointed him so much to die.

Frankie

by Terri de la Peña

She sits in stillness, her memory rekindled, recalling their friendship as a revolving series of photographic slides, linked by similarities, jolted by differences.

~

They had known each other since childhood, smashed piñatas together at birthday parties, giggled and played doctor in his parents' screened-in patio. Admiring her demure periwinkle gown, Frankie had even escorted her to the senior prom. She had teetered clumsily on high heels, envying the satin lapels and matching leg stripes of his grey tuxedo.

Two years later, when he revealed his decision to enter the Franciscan order, she whispered, "It won't work, Frankie."

"It beats getting shipped to Vietnam," he insisted. "I'll earn a B.A. so I can teach."

During their separation, she wrote to him often, sharing the unfolding trauma of her own life. When he left the Franciscans, he told her about his impending marriage.

"That won't work either," she responded in exasperation.

"I want *una familia* of my own. I'm not like you. I'm going to get a teaching job and settle down."

When his wife Cecilia had their baby boy, Frankie proudly pointed out the squalling dark-haired infant through the hospital viewing window.

"How could you do this, Frankie?"

"I'm happy now. And everything's going to be okay." He grinned, and she wanted to believe him.

Not long afterwards, she saw him in a gay bookstore in West Hollywood. "Frankie, it's starting."

"What? I'm just trying to buy your birthday present, *loca.*" His brown eyes avoided hers.

Some months later, she spied him among the sidewalk crowd at the

Gay Pride Parade. She waved, and impulsive Frankie trotted over to join her marching contingent.

"What will Cecilia say about this?" she asked while they strode side by side.

"She knows. I haven't been happy and..."

"Frankie, you have a wife who loves you, a darling *muchachito*..."

"Hey, I'm taking care of things. Everything'll be fine. I promise."

She looked at him, but did not answer.

With his divorce finalized, he introduced her to Lorenzo. She noticed the unfamiliar peacefulness in Frankie's manner, his constant smiles. She relaxed, knowing he was happy. Before that year ended, he died of AIDS.

~

Disconsolate, she sits with the other mourners in the quiet church. Thinking of his natural warmth, his constant hopefulness, she experiences a searing loss. Her lover, noting her glistening eyes and frequent sighs, squeezes her hand. But she cannot be comforted.

"I miss Frankie," she murmurs through her tears. She knows she always will.

Absalom

by Paul Attinello

(For Reid, who died)

I rest his head upon my lap,
brush back his hair wet from the grass,
weep quietly, and touch his cheeks,
his eyelids, mouth, the drying blood.

The sky goes on forever, blue
as angels' wings, shot through with white.
O Absalom, my son, my son.

The dusk pours darker blues downhill.
Arrange his passive hands, and cup
my own above his eyes, to catch
the last rays of a dying sun.

The doctors push me from the room.
I hear terse orders, painful moans,
the buzz of desperate machines.

Absalom, my son, my son,
would that I might die for you,
let me live no longer, but
walk blindly, weeping, into hell.

A smooth green hill, white flowers in
a quiet place, no birds, no clouds
out to the sunset's bloody sun.
I hold his body close and will not let it go.

O Absalom, my son, my son.

Fig Trees

by Ayofemi Folayan

"I'm a telephone hustler." He had declared it so proudly, with such confidence. "I'm not going to get no AIDS or no VD! I'm just going to give the best safe sex in town. My name's Chris." He barely paused between syllables.

I met him when we were both waiting to get tested at the Mandelker AIDS Clinic at the Gay and Lesbian Community Services Center. I was actually annoyed at his invasion of my privacy, and tried to bury myself in the pages of the *Lesbian News*, but Chris demanded my attention. He was wearing a fairly somber outfit for him: bright royal blue t-shirt, lavender pants, rainbow suspenders, red Converse high tops, and large chartreuse and orange parrot feather dangling from an ear cuff. He reminded me of my younger brother, David, who wore his hair in the same style, high flat-top Afro with the sides and back shaved down to the scalp.

I felt positively drab in one of the brightest outfits I own: a red, black and green dashiki and red slacks. I didn't want to talk to anyone, but this guy just kept rambling on. I hunched over my paper and turned my shoulder away from him with body language that clearly signalled, "Leave me alone." I looked up as the door to the clinic swung inward, afraid that someone I knew would recognize me. Despite my decision to have the antibody test, I was still somewhat embarrassed about the whole process. I slouched down even further behind the rectangular shield of newsprint and tried to stem the rising tide of anxiety I was feeling.

"I just came here from my therapy session." He shifted the accent of the word 'therapy' so it rhymed with 'happy.' "I'm hoping some day my therapist will finally get my head wrapped right." The tone of his voice revealed that he shared my nervousness. Without warning, he jumped up and bolted from the room. Right after that, the nurse called my name. Distracted by my own anxiety about the HIV test, I didn't give this guy another thought.

The next time I saw him, I was having breakfast at the Yukon

Mining Company. I was in a really foul mood that was not improving with the long wait for a table. I was just about to give up and search for a less crowded option, when he literally blew in the door, as the Santa Ana wind gave his wiry body a shove.

"Hi, sweetness."

I scowled as I looked up from perusing the latest issue of *The Vanguard,* but my facial muscles quickly relaxed as I looked into his deep brown eyes. On impulse I smiled.

"What's going on?" I was definitely more interested in his news.

Chris pointed outside to a gleaming grey Toyota truck, complete with paint detailing. "See my new toy?" he grinned. "Back in New York, everybody plays 'the numbers,' but here in L.A. my number is '9-7-6." He scanned the packed room and offered, "Wanna go somewhere else?" As I hesitated, he urged, "Oh, come on! Besides, I can give you a ride in my new truck." He brushed the sleeve of his grey velour jogging suit and commented, "See, it matches." On his head he had tied a hot pink bandanna.

Gallantly, he opened the door and helped me into the pristine black interior of the truck. I inhaled the rich new car smells and settled back against the bucket seat. Chris hopped in, fastened his seat belt and started the engine. "What's your pleasure?"

Half-joking I responded, "There's a really cool restaurant in Santa Barbara called Frimple's that has this huge tree growing right up through the middle of it. And they have terrific waffles!"

Chris put the truck into reverse and started to back out of the parking place.

"Whoa! What are you doing? We haven't even decided where we're going yet!" I protested.

"Frimple's sounds good to me. Besides, it will give me a chance to get some highway miles on this baby. Are you doing anything more important today?" And I really wasn't doing anything else, although my left brain was apoplectic at this departure from my careful, ordered practices. I was the woman who bought a pocket-sized datebook so I could have it with me even when I wasn't carrying a purse. I was the woman who scheduled appointments to wash my hand laundry or give myself a manicure. I was definitely not someone who would drive to

Santa Barbara on the spur of the moment. At least not before Chris.

Reluctantly I relinquished all the arguments that I was about to use against this unplanned adventure and agreed, "Not really. I have to meet someone around five o'clock."

"Great! I'll have you back to your car in plenty of time, I promise." Chris put a finger to his chest, tracing an "X" like a young child and affirmed, "Cross my heart and hope to die!" The phrase, echoing in my imagination, made me shudder.

"What's the matter, girl, are you cold?" His question reflected a tender quality that made me quite sentimental. He managed to reach behind my seat and pull out a scarlet sweater and turn down the air conditioning without sacrificing any control of his driving. Before I knew it, we were out on Highway 101, heading north. At the Topanga Canyon exit, Chris detoured into a drive-through long enough to get two orange juices and two hash browns "to tide us over."

I laughed so much I felt the muscles in my cheeks getting stronger from the effort. Chris was an ingenious storyteller, words skimming smoothly out of his mouth like polyurethane wheels on roller skates. The truck transported us along the highway so quietly it was almost as if we were floating on a magic carpet. Chris told me about growing up the youngest of four sons in Hawaii, where his father was stationed at Pearl Harbor. He had figured out that he was gay sometime after his junior year in high school, but he had waited until after graduation to leave home. "This can be an anniversary party," he joked. "I've been in Los Angeles three years this month." Other than coming out, his political consciousness was so far to the right of mine that my neck risked whiplash, but that didn't seem to interfere.

I knew that Chris was probably very good at his work. The unaffected way he told stories would easily translate into the relaxed and natural conversations that were necessary for successful phone sex.

"Chris?"

"Yeah, what is it?" He seemed to vibrate with excess energy as he guided the truck along the highway.

"Can I ask you something?" I hesitated.

"It all depends, sweetheart." He tightened the muscles around his mouth and waited for me to continue.

"I'm real curious about the phone sex. Will you tell me how it works?"

"I like you, okay? But some things just don't get talked about. Understand?

Feeling guilty, I nodded. I gulped and stared at my shoes in embarrassment. Chris reached out and grabbed my hand. He squeezed it, then brushed it against his mouth in a gentle kiss. Then he set it back in my lap where it had been. I looked out the window of the truck and noticed the sign indicating the turn-off to Port Hueneme. It was amazing what good time we had made.

Chris asked, "Which exit do I take?" as we came around the curve of the freeway into Santa Barbara. Only then did my stomach begin to growl in earnest complaint over the long-delayed breakfast.

At Frimple's, we waited for a table because Chris insisted on sitting right next to the enormous fig tree that climbed up from the floor. "I love trees, because they live a long time."

He was energetic and excited as he polished off his waffles and a side order of eggs and bacon. "Did you see the special on PBS about the giant redwood tree that they carved a tunnel through? They said it was at least a thousand years old!" As the server set the check on the table, he snatched it with his huge hand.

"No way! You drive all the way up here, the least I can do is pay for the meal!" I tugged at the limp slip of paper.

Chris looked at me with the patient expression usually reserved for frisky young puppies snapping frenetically at a forbidden object. "Get serious, girl. When I celebrate, it's on me." With that pronouncement, he slipped some bills from his wallet for the tip and stood up, signalling that he was ready to leave. "I promised I'd get you back in time for your meeting, so we'd better get going."

The last time I saw Chris was in November. I was coming out of the Center. We talked about my next reading at A Different Light bookstore in March. He promised to come this year. "I keep seeing your stuff all over the place, " he said. "Keep those cards and letters coming, girlfriend." He told me he had purchased a potted ficus, in honor of our trip to Frimple's. We didn't talk long, because he was on his way to his "thair-appy" session. As he walked away, I noticed how baggy the chocolate brown pants were, how gaunt and stark the features of his face. I didn't have to ask.

His roommate called me last week. Chris had made him promise to give me the ficus. I don't really have room for it in my tiny apartment, but I want to watch it grow up through my life, like the tree at Frimple's. Right after I hung up the phone, I heard on the news that a giant redwood crashed to the floor during the heavy rains the night before. The newscaster said it was estimated to be about twelve hundred years old. Now sunlight filters through that space in the forest where the massive tree had been.

The Go-Go Prince

by Eric Gutierrez

16 APRIL 1988

Last night I went to Disneyland with Mom and Dad, my aunt Cookie, uncle Reno and another of his girlfriends. Some special event for dentists and their families. I think we actually had fun but today, picturing myself riding the Matterhorn and wearing 3-D glasses while Michael Jackson moonwalks makes me feel ashamed. My brother and Turner didn't come with us as planned. Turner's in the hospital. I think we all know he has AIDS. No one seemed to want to own up to that knowledge, though. After dinner we huddled in a circle behind the Cadillac in the parking lot and prayed.

18 APRIL 1988

My brother asked me to meet him at their place after he gets off work and before he goes to the hospital (Kaiser, room 924B.) When he told me Turner has AIDS he couldn't look into my face. I had a hard time finding his, myself. He recited his news to the distant wall, interrupting his vow to do exactly as Turner wished in every regard, and breaking his own heart with a detail. "His eyes are so blue," he said.

16 MAY 1988

It's been, what, a month since Turner was diagnosed. Time passes and I've become so angry. My brother gives over to tears and hopelessness. They watch rented videos in bed and wait for death. We are all so afraid. What do I know of their life? And I can only suspect their terror. But I want to pierce flesh and crush stone thinking of those two hovering around the meager warmth of TV.

So what's it going to be? The Three Bears? Packey, the Runaway Pachyderm? Ali Baba and the 40 Thieves? Ok, I know, you don't have to tell me. You want to hear the tale of the Go-Go Prince.

It was known far and wide at a certain time that no one could do the twist like the Go-Go Prince. Or the Watusi, the Virginia Reel or the Hustle for that matter. The Go-Go Prince was quite simply the best, most joyous and splendiferous dancer the kingdom, the continent and world had ever seen. Pilgrimages were made by entire elfin tribes as well as by peasants and kings, not to mention the annual trek of the Association of Amalgamated Fishwives. Huge crowds took delight in watching him leap and spin and laugh in his purple cape and five-story platform shoes.

Well, one day the Go-Go Prince climbed from his bed and put on his platform shoes and cape but for some reason he couldn't dance. It didn't feel right, there was no joy. He stepped outside. Already gathered on his lawn were the pilgrims who had come to see him dance. He didn't want to disappoint the crowd but he knew there would be no dancing today. Time passed without so much as a toe tap from the Go-Go Prince and eventually the pilgrims stopped coming altogether.

One evening as the Go-Go Prince was climbing down from his shoes and preparing to go to bed, there was a knock on the cork to his home. He popped out the cork and standing before him was the Snake-Eyed Princess. "I be good! I be good!" he cried, fearing she had come to spank him. Now the Snake-Eyed Princess was the beautiful disciplinarian of the kingdom, a woman of unsurpassed beauty with two snake-heads where her eyes should have been.

"Relax," she said. The snakes surveyed the room. "I've come to ask you a question. Would you like to dance again?"

"I would love to love to dance again," cried the Go-Go Prince.

"Then you must do one thing," the Snake-Eyed Princess whispered.

"Tell me what I must do," begged the Go-Go Prince.

She pulled him closer so that the snakes' tongues flicked his eyelashes and said, "You must learn to dance even when there is no joy."

The Go-Go Prince drew back in horror. "I could never do that!" he cried. "Could I?"

The Snake-Eyed Princess drew her cloak about her and as she disappeared into the night she replied, "You're the Go-Go Prince."

22 MAY 1988

I think I have never been so proud of Mom and Dad as I have been this past month. No act for them has been too much, or too hard; nothing sickens them or beats them. Their pity and ego are gone for now and they work and live amid the cruellest fears. It's as if they had a third son.

26 JUNE 1988

Took the guys to see the movie, "Salsa." "Salsa: It's hot." Must admit, the billboard was intriguing but what a dog of a movie.

3 JULY 1988

The guys flew Delta to Hawaii this weekend. I went to a party and after an ideal day of paddling in a pool, mumbling in the sun, I was at peace, I thought, heading toward night. Suddenly, things hurt and it was a shapeless fear I had never felt before, a panic that my brother might die. Thinking now, it was the same feeling I had when I was three and lost at the market. It feels like you will never see home again.

7 SEPTEMBER 1988

My brother saw his doctor yesterday because his cold and chest congestion lingers. I pray to God he doesn't have pneumonia.

First thing in the morning the Go-Go Prince set off on the back of the wart hog the Snake-Eyed Princess had left tethered in the garden. His destination was the Unknown Territory. He was bound to learn something new in a place he had never been before. The first leap year he came upon some starving peasants enjoying a picnic of earth. They offered him a dirt clod and wished him well. The second leap year he met a one-legged frog who did a little jig in his honor. The third leap year he didn't see a soul. By the fourth leap year the Go-Go Prince was approaching the Unknown Territory. When he reached the river separating the world from the unknown, he saw Chongo the monkey, Elizabeth Kubler-Ross and a puppy head the size of a mush melon trying to undo the knot someone had tied in the current.

"It's impossible," shrieked Chongo.

"You're angry," said Kubler-Ross.

"No, I'm not," replied Chongo.

"Don't deny it, " said Kubler-Ross.

While Chongo and Kubler-Ross argued, the Go-Go Prince slid from the back of the wart hog and snuck across the temporarily dry river while the puppy head yipped and yapped from where it sat on its ears. The Go-Go Prince hadn't taken four steps into the Unknown Territory when he heard a voice that seemed to come from behind him.

"You, hey, you in the shoes. Come here."

He went back to the river bank but still couldn't see who had spoken.

"Down here," the voice yelled. Looking down, the Go-Go Prince could barely make out a tiny point on the ground.

"Do you know what you just did?" asked the Point.

"Nope," said the Go-Go Prince.

"You just passed the Point of No Return."

"I'm sorry, I didn't know. You were so tiny I just didn't see you."

"Not many do," explained the Point.

14 OCTOBER 1988

I'm starting from scratch, sitting in the doctor's waiting room, wanting lab tests to relieve sexual angst. T-cell count, syphilis test. Gonorrhea. What do I want from all of this?

29 OCTOBER 1988

I went to the Edelman Center for an AIDS test this morning. Tonight I'm going to see "Les Miserables."

12 NOVEMBER 1988

Negative negative negative negative. I ran around all day thanking God in every spare moment, even creating a few. All these years I've treated God like the Auto Club, never giving Him much thought but confident He would be there in an emergency. This year I've gone running back to the God of my childhood. I just don't seem to have the strength for secular humanism anymore.

7 MARCH 1989

I *invited my brother to lunch to apologize for having acted the physician the last time I saw him. Last week when we got together, he tried to choke down his food as I lectured on the evils to the immune system caused by alcohol and tobacco. A regular Carrie Nation. I suppose I shouldn't have been hurt or surprised when he cancelled out a half-hour before we were supposed to meet. I'm not present for him in the ways he needs me to be there. I just don't know how to love in a hands-off sort of way.*

The Point wanted to know what brought the Go-Go Prince to the Unknown Territory. When the Go-Go Prince had finished his tale, the Point was so moved he offered to turn the other way and let the Go-Go Prince return past the Point of No Return. The Go-Go Prince was very grateful for the offer but he refused. He had come too far, seen too much, to go back now. Not until he knew if it were possible to ever feel like dancing again. So he thanked the Point, stomped mud from his platforms, adjusted his cape on his shoulders and turned to the great Unknown.

As the Go-Go Prince disappeared into the horizon the Point whistled and cheered and clapped as hard as he could because he had never seen anyone march so bravely into the Unknown. The Point never stopped applauding for the Go-Go Prince even though he never saw him again. He continued to clap out a little rhythm just in case the Go-Go Prince could hear him and should feel like dancing. And in all the time to follow, the Point was certain there were days someone was doing the Charleston and the Merengue and the Jerk just beyond where the eye can see.

3 AUGUST 1989

Stopped by the guys' house and sat in the yard with them and their friends. I can't believe what a good time it was doing nothing.

31 OCTOBER 1989

Spoke with Turner on the phone today. He told me about a friend of his who grew tired of the needles, the tests, the fatigue, the diarrhea, the constant daily decision to fight and to live. "But people aren't willing to let someone choose to die," he said. If the phone were to ring now and the conversation start all over again I would find the voice to tell him that I'm people, that I am not ready to let him go, that I haven't loved him well enough yet, that I will need a little more time.

Excerpt from <u>Dead Cat: Do Not Open</u>

by David Moores

Dale was frowning at the whipped cream that topped his decaf cappucino. "Don't they know it's supposed to be frothy milk floating on top?" he fumed as he scooped it onto his plate. Once rid of the offending whipped cream he could start his story.

"I've learned a lot about AIDS because of what I went through with my best friend Bill. Bill died a year ago last June. It was almost three years after his diagnosis."

Jerry wasn't sure he wanted to hear, but he asked, "What happened to him?"

"Up until six months before he died he was pretty much normal. There were strange little things. I remember he had gotten a cactus needle stuck under his thumbnail when he was moving. It got infected; it was a fungus or something. His nailed turned color and looked real gross; he always kept a Band-aid on it. Until the day he died it never did heal."

"I never knew that," Sasha mused, "but now that you mention it, I remember seeing a Band-aid on his finger all the time." He held up his own thumb, contemplating an infection that would never go away.

Dale continued, "In October of last year Bill got a couple of small lesions on his face. It was a hard time for Bill. Up until then he could hide his disease from whomever he chose. More importantly he could hide it from himself. Now every time he looked in the mirror he had an ugly reminder of his own mortality. I don't think any of us really wants to deal with that issue."

He raised his eyebrows as he looked at Jerry and Sasha. Jerry shifted his weight uncomfortably in the chair as Dale went on.

"In April of last year Bill's ex-lover, Cory, took him to San Francisco for fun. While up there Bill began to have a hard time breathing. Cory wanted him to see a doctor up there but Bill said he'd wait til he got back to L.A. Bill could get free treatments at the VA hospital; he'd been an army medic in Vietnam. That's a whole 'nother story," Dale rolled his eyes. "I guess you get what you pay for. At least it was better than County General. Anyhow, as far as I know he had pneumonia, although no one ever said 'pneumocystis' to me. His lungs had filled with fluid either from the pneumonia or from possible lesions on his lungs. They weren't sure."

Jerry started to sweat and move nervously in his chair. Staring out the window his eyes locked on a large flashing sign across the street. WACKO WACKO it screamed in garish neon colors. He listened as Dale went on.

"They did a procedure to pump out the fluid that had built up in his lungs. That's what was making his breathing so difficult. After about five days they sent him home. They told him the fluid might build up again and if it did he'd have to come back for a repeat of the procedure."

Jerry suddenly noticed that his own breathing had become very shallow and he took several extra deep breaths to reassure himself that his lungs were still okay.

"About the first part of May Bill's mother come out from Missouri to stay with him. He was getting progressively weaker. He needed her help and I think they both sensed that they might not have a lot of time left to be together."

"I'm amazed how strong she was through it all," Sasha interrupted. "As tough as it was she treated us so well."

Jerry wondered where his mother was right now and if she would be there for him if he ended up like Bill. He knew better than to count on her.

"We had to take Bill back to the hospital because his lungs filled up again. This time they not only drained the fluid, but they sprayed the inside of his lungs with some kind of sealant. The doctor said that it might – he stressed the word 'might' – keep the fluid out of Bill's lungs. They still didn't know what was causing the fluid, but like a sinking ship taking on water his lungs had to be bailed out for Bill to stay afloat."

For the first time since he'd started this story Dale paused to consider how all of this might be affecting Jerry. To reassure Jerry that he wouldn't necessarily end up like Bill, Dale said, "One thing you have to remember, some of the treatment options used today didn't exist then. Besides, Bill chose to go the natural route – herbs and things like that. He weighed the toxic effects of the drugs and chemotherapy available and decided not to subject his body to it. He got into crystals, Chinese herbs, teas. I even remember him buying some oil that came from and Australian tree to rub on his lesions. I didn't always agree with his choices, but I supported him like I promised myself I would."

Jerry wasn't even sure of what treatment options there were for him to consider right now. He felt overloaded.

"The last time we took Bill to the hospital it was a Monday morning. His mom had called me and said he was having trouble breathing. He needed to go the the emergency room; could I take them out to the hospital. 'Of course,' I said.

"I was surprised at the hospital. They let both me and Bill's mother go into the emergency room with him. As we stood there separated from the other beds by thin curtains, I noticed blood dripping on the floor from the bed to our left. From behind the curtains to our right I heard nurses calling out a man's name trying to bring him back to consciousness. This room was definitely about life and death."

Jerry flashed on the one time he had been in an emergency room. He was about seven years old. He'd fallen from a tree and gashed his head. Blood was dripping everywhere, it was chaotic. He was crying, everyone else was screaming. In the end it only took four stitches to fix him up.

Dale relayed more details. "When the doctor arrived I stepped out in the hallway by the nurse's station. After about five minutes the doctor came out and explained to me that the choices were to send Bill upstairs to have the fluid drained off again, after which he could go back home again for another seven to ten days and then return to the hospital for a repeat procedure. With this the doctor might give him another six weeks. Or he could go home without the procedure and probably die within a week.

"It shocked me to hear that. I told the doctor that Bill deserved the truth and to please be very honest with him. We went back to Bill's bed. The doctor explained the options to Bill and his mother. I told Bill I would ask some questions for him. If he didn't want to hear the answers he should say so. I asked the doctor what would happen if Bill went home now. The doctor said eventually his lungs would fill. He would have a harder and harder time breathing. He would either suffocate or his heart would give out from the added strain."

Dale noticed Jerry's complexion pale.

"I know it sounds brutal. I just didn't think there should be any surprises and that Bill should have this information to make his decision. The doctor left us alone. I offered to leave too but Bill and his mother wanted me to stay and be a part of this. I asked Bill, 'What do you have left to do?' Bill knew what I meant. He answered, 'Nothing. I just want to go home and be comfortable.' It was settled that we would take him home and make his last days as comfortable as possible. We'd get a wheelchair, oxygen, whatever."

There was a break in the conversation as each man picked up his cappucino and contemplated the finality of Bill's decision. After a few minutes Jerry broke the silence. In a tentative voice he asked, "How did it go after you brought Bill home from the hospital that last time?"

Dale pushed his empty cup aside and went on. "We got a wheelchair from the hospital. By this time even with help Bill was too weak to walk. His mother and I managed to get him home and up two flights of stairs with no elevator. We got him settled in and I think he fell asleep for awhile.

"Later that Monday afternoon a large tank of oxygen was delivered. His mother and I were instructed how to use it. When Bill awoke we convinced him to try the oxygen. There was a clear plastic tube that hooked over his ears and under his nose where two smaller tubes delivered the oxygen to his nostrils. He hated it." Dale laughed, remembering how Bill would become obstinate, throw a tantrum and rip the tubes off his face.

"Maybe it was irritating?" Jerry speculated.

"I think it was more that he just hated being dependent on anything," Dale said and went on. "Cory, Bill's ex, came home and made some dinner for us. Bill, of course, didn't eat much. I stayed until about nine o'clock and then went home exhausted. Bill had gone to sleep and there wasn't much more to do. His mother spent the entire night in the chair next to Bill's bed, occasionally dozing off.

"Boy, Bill's mom was really there for him," Jerry said.

"She really was," Sasha agreed. "Bill needed her. She needed us. We became family."

Dale continued, "The next day, Tuesday, Sasha and I and some of Bill's other friends took turns sitting with him so his mother could get some rest. His brother flew in from New York that night. He and Bill hadn't seen each other in almost five years. I stayed until he arrived. He was younger than Bill but looked just like him. I went home and crashed. It had been two long days."

Sasha added, "It was a miracle that Bill's brother came when he did. At least they got to spend a little time together."

"So the next morning, Wednesday, I was sitting at home eating breakfast when the phone rang. It was Bill's mother. They had a little emergency, could I come over? Bill needed to have a bowel movement. He was too weak to get out of bed. She'd sent his brother to the drugstore to get a bedpan and whatever. I told her I'd be right over. In the meantime she called Steve, another of Bill's friends. He was there when I arrived. While waiting for Bill's brother to return from the drugstore I told Bill, 'Don't worry, if you have to shit, shit. We'll clean it up.' He held on.

"When his brother returned we decided to carry Bill to the toilet. I was shocked; his body was like a skeleton with thin tattered leprosy-like skin drawn over it. He had no strength left. He couldn't even wipe his own ass. Obviously what happened next was God working through me: I grabbed a couple of vinyl gloves, slipped them on and reached down and wiped Bill's ass for him. Believe me, that is not something I would choose or volunteer to do, but somebody had to do it. He was my best friend. I just did it."

"Geez!" Jerry exclaimed. He had a hard time imagining such helplessness.

"We got him cleaned up and back into bed. Steve told me he thought I was tougher than any Marine. I told everybody else to take a break out on the patio. They did and I sat with Bill.

"After a few minutes Bill looked up at me and said, 'Dale, I'm ready to go.' Earlier his mother and I had told him it was okay to let go if he wanted to. He didn't have to stay here for us." Dale smiled. "He lay there anticipating that something would happen. He was ready to die. Nothing happened. He looked up at me. I laughed as I said, 'Just like everything else, Bill, not in your time but in God's time. You just might be stuck here for awhile.' I was relieved to know he wasn't going to die just yet.

"His mother and brother came back in about twenty minutes. Steve had gone home. They suggested I take a break and get something to eat. It sounded like a good idea. I had a couple of errands to run too. As I stood in the doorway of Bill's bedroom I turned to Bill and said, 'Bye, babe, I'll see you later.'

"I ate, did my errands and when I returned to my place there was a message on my machine. Bill had died just ten minutes after I left. I immediately headed back to Bill's apartment. At the gate I picked up the security phone, and as I started to dial Bill's code I began to cry. Without finishing the code I hung up the phone and sat on the steps sobbing until Cory came around the corner. He had been called home from work. I dried my eyes and we went upstairs.

"It seemed with everyone's help things just went smoothly. Bill's mother told me she and his brother had been in the room talking and he had died shortly after I left. Bill's hands were cupped over his ears like this," Dale tilted his head slightly to the side and covered his ears with his cupped hands. "I think he was trying to block out the voices so it was easier to let go. The music he had asked me to put on before I left was playing when he died. It was called 'Astral Trip.' The one positive thing he'd said to me about dying was he'd get to see his grandmother, who he really liked.

"When the attendants from the mortuary arrived they handled everything normally. We'd gotten their number through AIDS Project Los Angeles, so they were AIDS-sensitive, thank God!

"I showed them where Bill was laying. One of them leaned over the bed to remove the oxygen tubes. I said, 'No, I'll do it.' I reached over and gently removed the tubes from behind his ears and under his nose. It was the last thing I did for my friend Bill."

Caring Without Answers

by Robin Podolsky

Alvaro had the face of an angel. When he stood, his shoulder blades poked out like vestigial wings.

We met on the day that I went to Chris Brownlie Hospice (CBH) as a volunteer. I had agreed to edit *Caregiver*, a publication of the AIDS Healthcare Foundation, which runs the Hospice. I felt that the job would be impossible without a closer connection to CBH. An experienced volunteer led me through the halls, introducing me to residents. I felt awkward as hell. I'm not at ease in situations when an outside imperative obligates me to befriend total strangers.

The first person that I met wanted, emphatically, to be left alone. The second was happily watching a TV screen which displayed nothing but snow. When we came to the room that Alvaro shared with his lover, Juan, he smiled warmly and invited me in. Of the two of us, I might have been the more grateful.

Juan and Alvaro were watching Spanish language news. Alvaro, it turned out, was ardent about Cuahtemoc Cardenas, the populist leader who may transform Mexican politics. Juan is from El Salvador. He came here for peace and quiet and a job. An hour after Alvaro's invitation, we were still talking and laughing.

Alvaro was twenty-five years old. Juan is almost forty. They met in Griffith Park, where they exchanged phone numbers and, as Alvaro says, "Nothing happened." Alvaro had given up on hearing from Juan when, two weeks later, he called and suggested a trip to the Azusa River. They became friends and then lovers. When Alvaro moved into the hospice from County/USC Hospital, they had been lovers for over two years.

"He loves me too much," whispered Alvaro one day. "When I go in the hospital and they tell me I have HIV, I say, if you want to go I understand. But he don't leave me. He come every day. Then I know how much he love me. Why else is he here? I don't have money. I don't have nothing but… me. He is my baby. *Mi amante.*"

Juan is a phlegmatic, habitually courteous man with a sudden vivid grin. When we met, he was in school, learning English and computer skills, looking for work and doting on Alvaro.

Juan connected with my lover, Janice, who also volunteered at the Hospice. Like Juan, Janice is a student and freshwater angler. They had a terrific time one night, talking irregular verbs, trout and What to Do After Graduation while Alvaro and I played cards with Janice's seven-year-old daughter.

I have never met anyone who could sustain the interest in television that Alvaro could. I can't remember a time in which he was awake and that machine wasn't on. Once, we were watching some *novela* (soap opera.) Alvaro had gone without speaking for so long that I wondered if courtesy kept him from saying that he felt like being alone. I had just made up my mind to leave when he gave me a look of such depthless sorrow that the world froze. *"No quiero morir,"* he told me. *"Quiero vivir.* You understand me?" A tear lined his cheek. "I don't want to die. I want to live." For once out of words, I took his hand.

Alvaro had shown me his driver's license, with its picture of his healthy self. His handsome face was not at all that of an angel then. Before his condition slipped, his mind teemed with questions about history, other countries and God.

In Juan, Alvaro had found the love of his life. He was a young man with all the pieces of a future who would leave nothing here but a tangle of love and loss in the hearts of his lover, his friends and the mother who would outlive him. I met her one night and learned where Alvaro got his sculpted features and voluble eyes.

He looked at me that afternoon with the defenseless eyes of a child and a young man's determined eyes and with the stunned wide-eyed stare of an old person who sees the shadow coming down. And the only answer I had was to witness his pain, to let it draw my own tears for as long as he needed me to.

There were more good times. Once, the four of us went out for

Salvadorian food. Then things began to change. Alvaro was vomiting more and talking less. My mother became seriously ill while my workload increased, and I found it much harder to visit the Hospice. When I tried to explain things to Alvaro, he told me that he understood, but between my lousy Spanish and his growing confusion, I'm not sure that he really did. I'm not sure.

Once, when Juan had left the room, Alvaro whispered, "I'm tired. If there is a drug that make me well, okay, but like this… I'm tired. But I'm afraid. I'm not afraid of my God, but I am afraid for *mi amante.* He always tell me 'you have to fight.' He love me too much."

"Let him love you now as much as he wants," I told him. "Later… he'll be okay."

That was our last serious conversation. I saw him a few more times, and then there came a period in which my list of things to do everyday began with my list of what hadn't gotten finished the day before. Finally, I had an afternoon to spend at Brownlie and interview Donna, the Hospice's bereavement counselor. Afterward, I thought, I could go and see Alvaro. The interview had begun on the outside patio, when Juan walked by. He came over and hugged me and then he said, "I tried to call you, but I can't find your phone number."

He watched my apprehension turn to certainty. "Nobody tell you? It happened Monday morning."

"What happened?" I demanded like an obstinate child. Donna said that Alvaro was dead. Juan nodded. He looked weary and tender and sad. "Are you going to be okay?" I asked him.

"Sure, sure…" he said gently. I wrote down our number for him. He took it and walked away.

Donna asked if I wanted to put off the interview until later. I assured her that I was perfectly fine and burst into tears. She held me, and then we got back to work.

Rain Dance

by Susan Silton

We ritualized the dog piss puddled on the floor of her studio above Main Street. The hallway where we circled the urinal shrine, with our heads flung back in uncontrollable laughter, was flooded by blue neon and the sallow moans of junkies shooting up in the alley below.

"Thank you, thank you God for this heavenly pee," I reached my hands towards the sky, testifying, my stomach aching from its exhaustive workout. Her pup, Jane, stared with bewilderment from another room.

"Bless you, Lord for giving us this circle of piss. We feel you here with us now, we feel you." She followed closely next to me, the nose earring and the crystal necklace bouncing in unison against her slight frame; in context I saw them as religious ornaments, mortal gifts to the gods on this sticky summer night. "Amen," I said, "Tell it, sister."

Our hands and feet cut the acrid air with sanctimonious motion; we wound our way around the stained wood floor with the feverish pitch of the blind, the deaf, and the diseased healed on TV. When the laughter finally died down that night in Dhana's stark hallway, I felt an edge of depression take hold, the kind that always seems to ride surreptitiously on the heels of a jubilant fit. We looked in each other's eyes, teary from hysteria, then down at the yellow pond whose pungency now left me weak and despairing.

"Well, it's getting pretty late. Do you want me to help you clean it up?" I asked politely, hoping her answer would be no. It was all now like a frightening dream; the horses on the merry-go-round first bobbing up and down gleefully and then suddenly the music becoming frantic as does the galloping pace of the hooves. I needed to wake up with fresh air and time alone. Just at that moment her AZT alarm went off.

"Oh boy, pill popping time," she said sarcastically. "No, I'll be fine, thanks, you go on," she responded, albeit distracted, to my question, and with that I was out her door and into the downtown night of the hookers and homeless, avoiding eye contact as I usually did here.

Three months later I am holding a pan under Dhana's trembling head, waiting for her to vomit for the second time in an hour. Light is a crack under the door and an annoying fluorescent bulb in the bathroom. Outside these colorless walls, faded from tirelessly housing the ill, the discomforted, the fearful and occasionally the grateful, footsteps canvas labyrinthine halls with a peculiar combination of calm and urgency. I hear the poised footfall of the nurses' routines. Like expectant mothers whose water has burst, they know the intervals and when to breathe.

One of my hands holds back her hair while the other tries to follow the lead of her head as it motions in half-light, groping for this to be over. I remember how I hated the smell of my own vomit as a child, there in the living room with the TV blaring. I'd run away hoping it would magically clean itself up, that there would be no physical evidence of my human fragility. Now, in a room reeking of vulnerability, we are both here, the one woman trusting the other, the other woman recalling the fetid living room but not running.

After a half-hour or so Dhana's nausea calms, or perhaps she's just too exhausted to even puke anymore. I help ease her fevered body down, sit on the edge of her bed and hold her sweaty hand, while she mumbles something half-deliriously about how disgusted I must be.

"Remember when Jane peed on your floor? And our little dance? God how funny that was," I whisper.

"That bitch," she says drowsily, the corners of her mouth forming a smile. "Jane. I love Jane," she trails and her head falls left, away from the room and from me, into sleep.

For a while I watch how her mouth drops and her eyes twitch though closed, and then I release her hand, take my coat and knapsack and listen to my own footsteps resounding through the quiet corridors after I've left her room. I take Third downtown, past cardboard houses lining Los Angeles Street, toward my loft across from the Flower Market, where at this hour, tulip and tuberose drift through the windows and briefly drown out the persistent odor of booze and grit. After I've had a chance to squeeze my cat, I reach for the Brazilian rain stick, filled with hundreds of seeds, and slowly turn it upside down to hear how rain can sound where no water exists. The rain dance is as much about faith as it is a call for cleansing. I lift the long, woven stick above my head and, imagining myself in the Amazon, painted and naked, I begin.

Excerpt from "The AIDS Dance"

by Rondo Mieczkowski

Enough?
It never comes.
There's always more to handle.
Hawks shadow the house.
Spiders clog the sugar bowl.
Wasps fall out of newspapers
their wet wings
spread to dry
ready to join their brothers
already swarming the house.

I smell something burning.
I've got a chill up my spine.
Did you hear something?
Do you smell gas?

I remember hearing/reading,
it was a long time ago,
that an army of lovers cannot be defeated.
It was
a long time ago.

My lovers are dying or dead now
but I can still feel their sperm in my body
curdling, rising
waking up
where is the moon?
the spirits of men

begin to hum
their wings clatter my bones
into the night
where are the stars?

I cannot see
I cannot hear
my senses throb
with the dead.

Justice, justice, justice,
the souls whisper.
My mind is an oven
snowy with heat
a train pulls up
shovels the bodies in
lovers twitch
get up
and begin their march
in the fire.

Someone defeated an army of lovers
hearts shattered on county wards.
Someone murdered a generation
wasting away from lack of sustenance.

Is this Dachau?
Is this Ethiopia?
Is this my own backyard?

As a child I only wanted
to play on the grass
be left alone

and watch the clouds.

Now lightning fucks the sky
ashes are raining down
where is the moon?
Justice, justice, justice,
the souls of my dead
sting their song
into my skin.
My flesh is burning off like,
my flesh is burning off like, like,
burning flesh.

Forget justice.
Forget the rules.
Forget fair play.
And forget what passes for innocence.

My lovers live in me
now
if you call this living.

Who can defeat
an army of the dead?

They only want
they only want
their revenge.

PART TWO

Testimonies

At Risk

by Gil Cuadros

It's just after Christmas
and the waiting room is filled
with artificial limbs,
bulbs that twinkle,
packages wrapped
empty as rattles.

I am slouched by the exit
and the X-mas cards
are taped to the wall,
horses in the snow,
doves in the air.
A Black woman scolds her boy
all nerves and cough.
She tells me it's the flu,
tugs at his rough collar,
patches of hair
are missing from his head.

He runs to touch the tree,
the balsa nativity,
the paint-chipped ornaments,
his face reflecting large and round.
To her, he breaks everything nice inside.
She threatens him
with a rolled up magazine,
an ancient *Life*

or a *Woman's Day*,
like my mother would read
and beat across my back,
poke me in the chest
till I hid far into the closet,
her dark dresses hanging over my head
and the promise of burning my hands
on top of the stove.

The boy's arms fly
covering his head and neck,
his small elbows
against her sharp paper.
She looks at me
and I look at my watch
knowing it's my appointed time,
I've been waiting all week for my results.
The nurse calls out my name
and the little boy thinks they want him.
He hugs his mother's leg.
She just pushes him off
with her other foot,
lynches him by the string
around his jacket's hood,
the windbreaker at his throat.

I am asked to wait inside the doctor's office
meant to impress with diplomas,
pictures of him and Tom Bradley,
the choking sound of an aquarium.
I am just like any other queer,

I've sucked down enough come
to know that I'm infected.
The doctor thumbs my folder,
looks like my father behind those glasses,
there's no reason for me to cry.
He runs his hands down my neck
live a lover, checking for swollen glands
and even with this he begins to wear gloves.
I nod when he says, "We assumed you would be."
The chair next to me is empty.

The doctor leads me through the corridor
to the reception area, where all hell breaks.
The little boy scatters underneath the seats
and scented branches.
She hunts him down with her nails
and the air is cracked
by the sound of her hands slapping
the boy's cheek.
I can hear her sucking teeth,
"Do you want me to get the belt?"
She knocks him down to the floor.
The boy refuses to cry, knowing
she can really give him something to cry about.
He doesn't give any lip.
The doctor moves on
to other patients, other rooms.
I didn't dare ask how long I've got,
palm over my mouth,
I say mother
softer than I ever did before.

The Garden

by Alan Zimmerman

I came home last night and more had been removed from the garden. More of *mine* had been removed to be *theirs*. The rocks and my ferns. For eleven years I've put in slips and twigs that became bushes and vines, places for my cats to climb in and hide under, all in a low light environment, 3'x50'. No one else was interested.

Then the people upstairs came in. The banana trees that protected me from the noise of the traffic were removed. And two boxwood trees and more – an orange tree.

They painted everything white, trampled the plants that didn't get paint on them and splattered the sidewalk. When I told them about tarps and my concern, I became the bad guy, the grouchy busybody.

Too many changes were taking place. I was being ignored. They sterilized all the existing character from the environment. My personal pots were rearranged; they suggested I paint my door and wall area. The toxic white, the dreaded killer of character, I being that character.

They were covert when necessary. When I would return home I'd discover three-foot sections of cannas and philodendrons missing. I'd find them in dumpster in the alley. I said if you want some space, leave the plants at my door so I can pot them, let's plan the garden, talk about it. I've been there a long time.

My fuchsia was killed by pruning, and Japanese maple. Then they cleared out the ground plants. They would say how much they liked something and next week it would be gone.

I began to plot revenge. Wanting to beat them at their own game, I started removing plants, hopefully the favorites they had left. You want it bare? I'll top it and show you bare. Some control. I found homes for the plants, moving them to friends' gardens for safety. It became a mission of preservation.

I ended up with a 3'x9' section. They ended up with forty feet of bare earth, and newly introduced baby tear clumps. I stared at the stark endless space defoliated with miniscule controlled mounds of green creeping their way tear by tear into my remaining bits of life.

This is all so scary, the gradual removal of me, the taking over by a foreign body that has no regard for me. This is what AIDS is. Each new symptom, each inch that gets lost to a lesion, each part contaminated by a virus with its own ideas, means my defense system is that much more ineffective. Inch by inch. I see it as dying. Being dwindled away, in front of my eyes, into a sterile non-entity. Newly pulled plants lying limp, shriveling from life.

A week ago they planted full grown zinnias. Then asked with pride, how do you like them?

Last night I stepped on a zinnia. I stormed up and down the walk a few times and then I just stomped on a zinnia. Smashed and broke it to bits. I already had imagined them not making it, mildewing for lack of sun, but I had to take an active part in the demise of the fruits of their labors. Not let them take over so easily. Remind them that someone is still here and not content to sit still.

I woke up early this morning with anticipation and looked out a window in the direction of the scene of the crime, the vegecide, to see if something out there was glaring, just waiting for my return. Aha! He looked in the direction of the demised zinnia, obviously guilty! Or maybe, looking out there in the early light, a strange glow would be etched in the air, the very spot where the poor flower had so wantonly been sacrificed. I wasn't even aware of its color.

And still the virus creeps.

If I can't grow along one path, the universe pulls up my roots and I replant in another direction. If something doesn't work, find something that will. With every gain a little is lost and except for one zinnia, life goes on. But even one flower's death diminishes me.

Ave

by Paul Attinello

I am, on the whole, allergic to Christianity. Even when dealing with illness, fear or unexpected levels of despair, I instinctively avoid anything with God's name on it. Prayer and spirituality, particularly with Bible quotations and personal relationships with Jesus plastered all over them, leave me cold with distaste. Since I am a classical singer, and one of my less stressful ways of making money is singing in churches, this sometimes leaves me in an awkward position. I avoid jobs that put me in front of the congregation, where I must pretend to pay attention, and prefer isolated balconies in the back where I can be secular and read. Singing in Latin helps. Sometimes, though, at the height of a Christmas mass or in the midst of an exceptional, sincerely reverent piece of music, I can understand the attraction of the whole business.

A year or so ago, maybe longer, I was driving on the freeway, listening to a tape of motets by Josquin. An 'Ave Maria' came on, a late work, one of his most famous. The text is the usual one, full of 'nos' and 'nostros' – we, us; phrases like 'deliver us,' 'intercede for us.' At the very end, though, Josquin alters the traditional text (which must have caused a scandal in the sixteenth century): the counterpoint freezes, and all the voices join in deadly serious chords, singing: 'O mater Dei, memento mei.' Mother of God, remember me. Me, not us. Like the hook at the end of a business letter: I hope to hear from you soon, I anxiously await your reply. Thank you so much for your kind attention.

Merciful one, the loving mother. I had had a rough week, newly sick with AZT, out of a job, desperate about the rent, watching my T-cell count drift into the danger zone. I heard the end of that motet, and started playing it over and over: backing up past the last minute or so, hearing those final words, hitting the off switch, driving for a bit, turning it on again. The tape was starting to sound strange, the cheap tape deck was stretching and damaging it from too many repetitions. Mother of God, remember me. I realized that this was getting dangerous, that I would either have to pull the car over or stop crying so hard. Mother of God, remember *me.*

It must have been six or eight months later that I went home for Christmas, determined to tell my family about what is obliquely called my 'health status.' My father already knew, and was sympathetic, in his gentle, kindly, rather anesthetized way. I had spent the previous three months – not figuring out different ways of telling them, as I should have – but wishing it would all stop, go away, somehow become unnecessary, and I avoided any plan or thought about the coming confrontation. So I went home to the cold East, looking terrible – my face raw, red with psoriasis, my increasingly fragile digestion dreading the prospect of holiday food, and of course I caught some sort of flu for the first five days.

Three or four nights after Christmas, a couple of days before my plane was to leave, all of the adults were, for once, together at the dinner table, lingering over dessert; both of my nieces had gone downstairs to watch television. Some distant relatives of my sister-in-law, who had never met our family, were supposed to come by in about half an hour to chat and meet everybody. I asked everyone to pay attention for a moment, as I had something important to tell them. My father tried to stop me, but he was, as always, easy to override. So I told them, voice shaking, wishing I were dead already, wishing everything would just stop.

The reactions varied, but those of the women were all moments I do not expect to forget. My eldest sister, looking utterly sympathetic, asked if there was anything, anything at all, that she could do for me. She sounded and looked so wise and kind at that moment, it nearly made me calm; I think I loved her then as I hadn't for years, since she was my best friend in the world, before she turned away to get married. My sister-in-law, a sweet but sensitive woman with a midwestern fundamentalist background, burst into tears and said: "It just didn't need to happen." I knew what that meant, and wasn't pleased; but she had good intentions, and didn't elaborate. She has been kind enough not to say since then what she implied that evening, that I never should have been gay, or never should have been promiscuous, or something.

But before either of them said anything, my mother reacted. "I knew it." That was all, in that sharp, anguished tone that is so familiar, that resonates through so much of my memory – at least those parts of my memory that are still intact, even in the spots when there are no words left, no memory of what was said in that awful tone. No sympathy, nothing.

My mind wasn't exactly reacting to any of this, just filing it for later, when I would return to California and recover. When I would watch the mental videotape one frame at a time, freezing moments, and turning it off at the worst points, like a fascinating horror film that you can't quite bear to watch.

Then, of course, we had to clean up and greet our new guests, who were nice Southern folks in a cheerful mood. The family managed quite well, chatting, serving food and drinks, showing vacation slides, acting pleasant and entertained. When they were gone, everyone cleaned up, distant, quiet, struggling with various emotions and unwilling to discuss them. As usual, the difficulty of predicting or managing my mother's reaction froze us all. Our central concern at this time. At all times.

Later, when I went to bed – it was early, but I was exhausted – she came in her robe and sat by me on the bed. She was kinder, and wanted to talk. The first thing she said was, "I know this must be hard for you too." I was paying attention to her later words, trying to answer questions and respond with the typical reassurances, emphasize that everything was really fine, that there was nothing to worry about, and so on; but a part of my mind was already chewing over this line, amazed by its implications. I am so disfigured that I loathe, I fear, seeing people. I have just come thousands of miles to catch the flu, which I knew I could not avoid. The man I love most died seven years ago, died bloated and hideous and in pain; I remember too many people who are dead; I am taking a medicine that makes me so sick I don't want to get up in the morning; I don't know what will happen to me, or how painful or expensive or protracted it might be. I don't even know how to be terrified, I'm just numb. "I know this must be hard for you too."

A few months later, my younger sister visited me while on a business trip. Among her various lectures, she complained that I had frightened everyone by looking so terrible when I came home for Christmas, that I should not allow myself to look so sick. I listened to her plans and advice, her elaborate critiques of my career and personal habits, but now I had another idea to chew over in secret, and become amazed at the mental processes it suggested.

I know they love me, I mean they really love me. I am closer to my mother than anyone on earth, although too much of our time together has been caught up in a gray, dead place just previous to rage and hatred, where we tensely analyze each other's sentences for attacks or abandonments. We mirror each other, and are helpless in the grip of our emotions – but they're not even our emotions: the emotions we inherited, the ones we can't possibly understand. She must have nightmares that resemble mine, deserted cities, fields of broken ice, bloodied feet, she should be pitied, but still. I hate writing this, I hate saying this, I know that somehow, before or after my death, someone will give this to her, and it will hurt her deeply. And yet I need for her to know about me, I want her to know who I really am, and I am caught in the ancient trap of parents – I don't dare be too honest, I don't want to hurt them too deeply, but I am strangling, choking on so many things I can't say. But this is who I am, I don't have time to hide anymore, I don't have any time left to be silent.

I know this must be hard for you, too.

Mother of God – remember me?

The Waiting Room

by Crespin Rosas

Blond and already butch, Timmy Miller screamed at the top of his lungs as he was dragged by the ear to the principal's office. He resisted arrest with more common knowledge of profanity than any of his peers. "What I do? What I do? Dammit, what the hell did I do?" he howled, his face as red as a Hawaiian Punch mustache.

His profanity captivated me, the small timid pretty boy who wanted to be more the brute. I admired his roughness, along with the blond shimmering hair floating up from his head in a cowlick as he was carried away.

Once during a math test, I attempted such bravery, letting my eyes wander to Mark Schwartz's paper. Miss Charmichael's eagle eyes caught me through her thick Coke bottle glasses. "If anyone is caught sharing answers they will be sent to the principal's office and receive and automatic 'F.'" The thought of an 'F' was terrifying, but no less frightening was the prospect of being sent to Sister Marie.

The day Miss Charmichael dragged Timmy away she sported one of her infamous identical-patterned outfits, the color of which was brick-red with large white polka dots. Its shape hung on her like the Liberty Bell. Atop her head Miss Charmichael wore a matching Minnie Mouse bow in her henna-red hair. I imagined her hanging from the top of a belfry, her long scraggly legs sounding out against her dress – " Ding, dong, ding" – as she dragged Timmy down the hall to Sister Marie's office.

Timmy had cheated on tests before and he was good at it, too. He had been sent to the principal's office time and time again, but never for cheating. Timmy was always such a little punk; I used to have the biggest crush on him when I was a kid.

~

I had never taken the AIDS test before. When I was checking in at the doctor's office the nurse handed me a questionnaire. At the top of the page was a space for a fictitious name. I handed the form back to her, pointing to the blank space. "It's okay," I said, "I don't mind using my real name."

"No, you don't understand," she told me. "You have to have a fictitious name."

Names pummeled the inside of my head: John Doe, Larry Smith, Ivan Crumb. If anything bad was going to happen it was going to happen to Ivan, Joe, or Larry. Then an inspiration came to me and I filled in a name at the top of the page... age 22.

Later in the doctor's office we went over the answers orally. I felt as I were telling the good old doctor about my masturbations, with whom and what I thought about while I was doing it. How often do I have sex? Did I use protection? Was I passive or aggressive?

Well, the truth is I hardly ever had sex. Depending on whether I was in love or not at the time determined when I was passive or aggressive and if I used protection.

"It's okay," he told me, "These questions are simply routine. This is all confidential and strictly for your medical benefit."

I was given an information booklet – *From Your Navel to Your Knees* – explaining the disease and its symptoms, its conditions and of course, the possibilities. I was so exhausted and dazed from these events that I barely noticed when a long rubber tube was tightened around my arm.

If there's one thing I cannot stand, it's giving blood. The thought of my life's blood flow being tapped is nauseating. What if there was an emergency? What if for some reason the nurse left the room and never came back? I knew I wouldn't have the courage to remove the needle myself, and I would end up a bloodless corpse.

After extracting two vials of blood the needle was removed. A bruise began to appear around the small puncture wound but was covered with a wet sterile cotton ball by the glove-protected nurse. I made arrangements with the receptionist to return in two weeks' time. I left with his advice in my ears: "Not to worry – just because your HIV test may be positive does not mean you have AIDS."

~

Miss Charmichael would leave Timmy sitting in the hall outside Sister Marie's office. "Now you just sit here and wait, young man, and in the meantime just think about what you've done!"

When class was over I would walk by him in the hall and he would still be waiting. She always made him sit awhile to let him contemplate his fate.

Staring down at him from the walls was a statue of our crucified Christ, a circle of thorns around his head with droplets of red paint protruding from prickly spears. On the opposite side of the statue were the Stations of the Cross. Since they were the only things in the room besides himself, they were the only things for him to think about. She would make him sit on the hard, cold bench and wait an eternity before calling his name.

~

Two weeks later when I return to the doctor's office I notice there are other people waiting. I do not remember there being anyone else before. I sign in and take a seat. Across from me a handsome young man looks up from his magazine and smiles. I want to ask him if he knows what he's doing. I want to scream at him and say, "Do you know where you are? Do you know why I'm here?" Instead I look down and close my eyes.

There is not very much to do while waiting for the nurse to call me. I look over a few magazines – *Palm Springs Life, Travel & Leisure, Town and Country*, and it makes me wonder: how much are doctors really making off this disease anyway? I close my eyes again, trying to escape my thoughts, but all I can see is the man across from me smiling. All I can see are men's smiles.

How many smiles could be inside me, eating me away? How many smiles could have been deadly and how many have I turned away from?

All of a sudden the nurse interrupts, calling my fictitious name. In that moment it's as if I'm somewhere else listening to a small forgotten voice.

"It's no sweat," Timmy says, his voice so small only because I've grown so much older. "You'll get through it; I always did!"

"Timmy," I say, "I'm not like you." He gives me a look as if I've made some great mistake. "It's not the same! This isn't third grade anymore!"

"Sure it is! You're in the third grade for the rest of your life. Sometimes you get away with things, sometimes you don't."

Before I can say another word the nurse calls out again, "Timmy Miller?"

I look at Timmy, half-expecting a punch if I don't go in. But he just sits there, swinging his legs above the floor, his blond hair and blue eyes patient, waiting for Sister Marie.

40

by Paul Monette

oh boy oh boy four years to go before
Robert Louis Stevenson dies in Samoa
gimme four more and I'll get a degree
in Greek statues I'll learn Chinese be kind
to my dearest enemies lady lady
save us a dance it's coming down in sheets
out there rivers of frangipani white
clouded peaks the cold volcanoes oh please
be kind to us who are not kidnapped save
by demons we father forth 40's half
a death these days World War I all over
the flower of a generation gone
to bits in Flanders like a rugby match
gone haywire all the poets gunned and buttered
till only Shaw was left to grow up and
Rebecca West grew barren as the wives
of ancient Thebes and life sucked no more tea
look the UN is 40 and solves nothing
and I saw day ten weeks after the light
show at Hiroshima and also solved
nothing ask any phobic it's not the heights
it's the edges that get you that weird thing
of being drawn to the precipice do it
the time has come to take the plunge and none
of your youthly coy and basket shots will
save you time doesn't give a fuck oh but
we planned such plans if the war hadn't come

~ 40 ~

and the weather had held and life had cleared
like a late Manet the scot died half a world
from the cinder choke of his native damp
and so will I bone-thin and sunburned blown
like a sailor take my slot in the coral
chambers still if I must be me not him
no buccaneer silver Jekyll and Hyde
to make me fit for a boy to read if I
must go early give me please one friend one
year but nothing's enough and the cliffs at Thera
where the old world ended tomorrow my love
is a stolen kiss but we sail together
if we sail at all hey 40's kid stuff

PART THREE

Tales

Excerpt from "D.O.A."

by Keith Antar Mason

i am a straight pin prince
i am a gran zombi
and they want
they want
they want to drain
my blood... i am a green monkey
curse... i am haitian
born on the island of circe

... if you see me walking down
the street and I start
to cry each time we meet
walk on by...

in black america
righteous black america
i die a lone still
a shamed
of who i am
of who i love

the huxtables would not take me in
in my family blood now
is the crisis
a young man with no job
enlisting to get
out

i learn the truth
i learn
the way of voodoo priests
i am a zombi
my blood
is my history
and i learn

that this is the only
way for me to come out positive

i loved the way the girlies
used to say
he is so fine…
he
is so cute

and we slept

to gather

in rock houses
to keep the pipe
lit   to blow the pipe
residue dreams into
our souls

i learned from the doctor
while enlisting
that i got it
that i got death for a cousin
a homeboy   best friend

... if you see me walking down
the street and I start
to cry each time we meet
walk on by...

and the huxtables did not take me in
they think i am gay
they think that i deserve this
i was a junkie
a gangbanger
and they gave up on me
in righteous america
i will die alone
and they want to erase
my name from the temple walls
in Luxor
and not remember me

not remember that they sentenced
me to death by silence
by denial

i am a straight pin prince
pharaoh's son
a gran zombi

... if you see me walking down
the street and i start to cry......

Excerpt from "Vigil/Manifesto," a solo performance work

by Tim Miller

For the week of the AIDS Coalition to Unleash Power (ACT UP/LA) Vigil at L.A. County General Hospital where the freeways meet in Beautiful East L.A. We're here to demand proper care, programs and an AIDS ward here at the biggest hospital in the world.

There is a big building behind me
a very big building
and on this building these words are written:

"Erected by the citizens of the County of Los Angeles to provide hospital care for the acutely ill and suffering to whom the doctors of the attending staff give their services without charge in order that no citizen of the County shall be deprived of health or lack of life for lack of such care and services."

There is a big building behind me.
It has angels and hunky laborers and those words carved onto it. I looked up at these words this morning after waking up on the cold cement and going to the bathroom by the perpetually blood-stained walls of the public toilet.
Why do those words sound so old and crinkly,
like they just slithered off some asshole's Victrola?

Have the County Board of Supervisors, or the Mayor, or the Governor, or the fucking President ever read those words? Which were chiseled in during the administration of Herbert Hoover, *that tacky queen!*
Oops! Sorry, Herb.
I got you mixed up with your girlfriend, J. Edgar.

And lots of us have been gathered here this week to try to make those words become true.

As I sat on the beach on Inauguration Day, the day before this vigil began, I sat in Venice near the homo/zone AKA Speedo/Lido, three things happened:

I saw the jet airplanes taking off from LAX and I thought of my recent and brutal fear of flying, and about Elizabeth Marek who died in the bombing of Flight 103 in Scotland. She was from here, in Venice Beach, and was a spectacular lesbian and performer and peace activist who got blown up at 33,000 feet.
No conclusions here, just a little context.

I watched the planes taking off over the Pacific Ocean, and on the beach arrives a Midwestern tourist family, shooting lotsa pictures to be sent back to Hays, Kansas with the caption, "Here we are on the Beach in January!!!" This group includes a mother-type who shouts to the others very loud, "I don't care what any of you want, I have no interest in going to Mexico!"

And then I hear an announcement over the loudspeaker on the lifeguard's truck which says, "Attention! All Lifeguards! Begin checking all persons laying in the sun to see if any of them are a dead body!"

This is the world I am living in, this day in front of County General Hospital.

There is a building, there is a big building
There is a big building on the hill behind me
and something has been happening here
in front of this building
people have passed seven days and seven nights in front of this building together... soup has been made... stories been told... performances been done... TV cameras been pointed... wet sloppy noisy sex been had by those two perseverent dudes in that pup tent over there... wobbling and shaking... and I say unto you now that if Boy Scouts had been like this I might have made it past Tenderfoot.

...gestures have been made... sleeping on the pavement...in the cold and the rain... and most intense of all... we in ACT UP/LA have seen what each other looks like before coffee in the morning... and yet still we are here... because demands have been made... demands to this City, County, State and Country to help our people live...

Now, what has actually happened here?
Has all this stuff made County General Hospital rise from its foundations and fly away,
trailing rotten plumbing, sadnesses, and a thousand IV tubes
doing a slow anti-viral drip as it disappears over the barrio?

No, that has not happened.

But maybe it will make some other things happen:

Like maybe when the County gets its shit together, people who are dealing with AIDS stuff right now and don't have health insurance will have a place to go where they won't have to sit in a public hallway on a hard bench getting their chemo and throwing up from the side effects in view of all

Like maybe it will begin to seem to more of us that it is at least as important to get proper health care ASAP to people who need it as it is to shop for a new leather jacket or to make yet another performance piece which obliquely deconstructs print advertising, and believe me, I've made my share of those

Like maybe a new kind of community is being born

Like maybe sleeping outside here in East L.A. has stretched a few of us to think in a real way what it is like for the 80,000 people who will sleep in cardboard boxes in this City of Angels tonight, some of whom have gathered here with us, walked the four miles from Skid Row, shared some food and found a safer place to sleep through the night

Like maybe this is a whole new cultural time arriving, of people gathered around a bunch of votive candles trying to tell each other a coupla'

stories waiting for morning to come

Like maybe we fags and lesbos can become a model for how Americans can stop forgetting and holding in and avoiding and feeding off of a lot of suffering in this world and off the world herself as she strains to deal with my 1974 Gremlin's carbon dioxide

Like maybe next time we won't be electing the country club trustee President of the United States and believe me, there is waltzing in Washington right now

Like maybe it is time for lines to be drawn, some absolutes to be acknowledged, some choices to be made

Because, because, because...

Because silence actually does equal death.

Because action actually does equal life.
These are not metaphors, or gym wear.

Because there may not be all that much time left.

Because my strongest art- and life-filled moment last year was a civil disobedience action in front of the Federal Building in L.A. And with each drawn outline of a friend dead from AIDS on the pavement, pure spectacle was happening, drums were beating, hearts were pounding, hands and bodies covered and gritty with chalk, trying to make the big picture, which more and more seems to be the one that matters most to me.

Because maybe any function of art, commerce or spiritualism that does not basically work in some kind of direction toward healing the sick, fostering communication, easing suffering, feeding bodies or saving the planet just ought to get back to a Reaganesque 1980 where it would be much more comfortable.

Because maybe it's time for a lot of art to be quite useful.

Because maybe it's not enough for us to be sad and pissed off for our boyfriends or our friends who are boys who have been lost to us; there are lots different kinds of people there in that building behind me.

Because last month I walked around the border near Tijuana with my friend Guillermo who told me that on that square mile more people die each year than on any other place in North America – run over by cars crossing the border, asphyxiated in the trunks of automobiles, or shot by crazed North San Diego County lunatics. I know this is just one injustice out of a zillion, but it cannot be foreign to us. This cannot be ignored. It's in out pockets, it's in our bed, it is next door to Sea World amusement park. Shamu the dancing killer whale is watching us to see if we can hook up, we homos, people of color, the undocumented, feminist ecologists, crazed global performance artists, *and all of you straight white guys too, both of you!*

Because some part of us is smoldering in our spirits and our actions into a way for a future to be built from this thing North Americans need to learn about pain and suffering and loss.

Because each of us – writing, agitating, painting, kissing, performing, designing, activating, fellating, detailing, coiffing, public relating, primping, obsessing, committing, masturbating – might make a society not quite so stuck on itself and able to speak so fucking glibly about kindness and gentleness!

Because there's no question that more lesbian peace activists from Venice will be blown out of the sky over Lockerbie or Burbank.

Because there's no question, each of us is going to have to go to someplace like Mexico.

Because there's no question, each of us is going to have to walk along the beach and find a body or two, there in the sand.

The Surreal Answer the World Hands You

by Aleida Rodríguez

"If there is a heaven, this is it."
– Michael Callen, AIDS survivor and activist

I called up Ricardo's doctor to find out how the tests came out and he lowered his voice apologetically and said: He's got thrush. Thrush! The name of an innocuous bird and also the enemy of the Man from U.N.C.L.E. This is the surreal answer the world hands you. And though there's a lozenge he can dissolve under his tongue to kill the candida fungus, I can't help feeling this is the first step in the spiral down. The other morning he woke me up with a litany of complaints: My chest hurts; I can't breathe; I have a fever. So, though it was twenty to six, I got up and fetched him something to drink and an aspirin. Then he said: I'm scared. So I held him, and he said, after a little bit: I'm such a ninny. But I said: Just shut up and let me hold you. And he fell back asleep. I still had a few minutes before I had to get up for work, so I dozed. If I had been asleep it would've been a dream, but I was just barely under, so it was a picture projected on a very thin screen: There was a two-lane highway winding along the base of some mountains, and there was a guy, not me, driving alone in a sports car with the top down – though it was very cold, not snowing, but cold. Next to him on the seat was a rifle he had just fired into the dense forest on one side of the road. Big Foot had been rustling in those trees, but there was no indication he meant the man any harm. Maybe he was just trying to make contact, you know? But the guy thinks: Great, I've scared him off, maybe I've even winged him. And he continues driving north. But who knows if the guy didn't fuck things up completely by having fired at him? What do you *mean* what's Big Foot for me? He's *death*, of course. He's *my* death and the death of those I *love* and he's incomprehensible! And, yes, I haven't wanted to meet him, or even look at him, and I've sniped at him to keep him away. And maybe now I've fucked things up completely. The next day Ricardo was back to his usual self, all peppy and with no memory of what he'd felt the night before. His fever had gone down, and he was sweating freely. And when I asked him where his *orishas* had been when he'd needed them, he got angry and said he hadn't really been that afraid, he'd just been half-asleep and hadn't meant it. And I allow myself to get jerked around by how he feels and what he says – and I can't afford to do that. I have to be prepared. I can't forget about everything just because he feels OK today. The other day I was working at my computer, writing about my fear of Ricardo's death, and suddenly, through an open window, I saw a couple of ravens swooping and darting, just swooping and darting, and I immediately switched channels and started writing about *them*. But it was a little scary, you know? Something or someone came over me and took over the controls: We control the vertical; we control the horizontal. Yeah, I know, there's an answer in there somewhere, but it's too transcended for me to be able to make any use of it right now. I'm too terrified to recognize what those birds were trying to tell me.

Excerpts from "Things to Do"

by Paul Decker

NINE

Bruce was right and Bruce was wrong. It turned out all sorts of guys wanted to meet Allen after his little camping excursion, but all of them were married. But they invited him to parties that Allen went to, because maybe that's where Mr. Right might be hiding and if he didn't go, he'd never meet him, but it seemed like all Allen ever met were more couples that thought he was "incredibly entertaining." Allen was flattered when smartly graying bankers and lawyers who steered political committees and still had good bodies told him, "Los Angeles is so full of bimbos, it's refreshing to meet someone so young and cute who is so smart and funny," until he realized what they really meant was "Oooooh! Fresh Meat!" Allen didn't have the heart to tell them the reason he was so smart and funny was because he was over thirty and only *looked* like a child.

So the married people invited him to more parties where he met more couples, and everyone thought he was charming but a bit aloof, which he was, because dating was crummy enough without falling in love with married men. Allen noticed if there happened to be other singles at these parties they wouldn't talk to him – if they were young they thought Allen was their age and therefore competition, and if they were older they thought Allen was hustling, since he was young and cute and unattached. So no one ever went home with him.

The couple who invited him over the most was Dick and Dick, two lovers who were known to their friends as Big Dick and Little Dick, because one was tall and muscled and gorgeous, and the other was thin and slight and sort of blah. Allen couldn't bring himself to call them Big Dick and Little Dick to their faces, however, since after seeing them in their Speedos at a pool party it became quite apparent (and rather ironic) that their nicknames should have been reversed. No one would ever tell Allen who had dubbed them Big D and Little D, but Allen suspected it was Big Dick himself, perhaps to throw suspicion off his shortcomings.

Allen had met the Dicks, who turned out to be relatively fun despite being bankers, on his camping trip from Hell, but whenever he went to their house he would find himself trapped in a land of chinos and power ties not of his own design. Allen tried to make the usual cocktail party chatter, but found that since he didn't own a house, a personal computer, or stocks and bonds of any kind, the only question he could ask or answer as, "So, who do you know, Big Dick or Little Dick?" (It seemed they were a rather independent couple and few people actually knew them both.) Allen found this line of conversation increasingly amusing, because he barely knew either, but everyone *he* asked had the same answer: "Oh, (Big or Little) Dick and I used to date for awhile."

Allen finally figured out that this was L.A. lingo for, "We used to fuck," or, more likely, "We only tricked once, but I have money and he makes a fabulous brunch so we still network." Allen absolutely *refused* to "network" since he had figured out it was a euphemism for "hitting people up you don't know for favors you haven't earned," so to keep the conversation going he blurted out, sort of by accident, "Well, I guess I'm the only one at this party who hasn't had sex with one of the hosts!" at which point the entire party stopped cold. When Allen was excited or drunk or even sometimes just being clever, his voice could really carry.

Luckily, Little Dick grabbed his arm and led him away from the stupefied crowd, announcing, "Well, we can fix *that* soon enough!" but since Little Dick was extremely drunk and definitely not the half of the couple Allen thought was attractive (even though this had changed somewhat once Allen got a load of Little Dick in his Speedo), Allen just giggled and maneuvered his way into the bathroom. This being the Hollywood Hills, the bathroom had a sliding glass door that opened onto the pool, which gave Allen a back exit through which to disappear into the night.

Once home, Allen wondered why, if the only thing those people could talk about was money, and all those people had sex but were so fucked up they refused to admit it, and all those people had to get drunk before they could even *flirt,* why was *he* the one home alone with the cats at 11:15 on a Saturday night?

Allen decided maybe he'd better start wearing chinos.

TWENTY-ONE

Allen had always thought that Big Dick was good-looking in a strapping, Midwestern kind of way, and certainly much better looking than Little Dick, but he never thought Big Dick was actually *sexy.* He was married for one thing, which made him off-limits, and he was married to a real dip, for another. Allen always figured if Big Dick was into Little Dick, he must be a closet dullard. So aside from a few reciprocal parties, he and Big Dick stayed only in casual contact, even though they lived just a few minutes from each other, Big Dick on the right side of the hills, Allen on the wrong.

But now Big Dick had called Allen out of the blue and told him that he and Little Dick were drifting apart, and he was actually laughing about it. Breaking up with his drunken lover after eight years had actually made Big Dick funny. And button-down Big Dick, now that he cracked jokes and loosened up a little, suddenly had become *very sexy.* And Big Dick had obviously been sublimating a lot of sexual energy at the gym, because his body, which used to be nice, was now more along the lines of incredible. He was bigger, bulkier, beefier, and towered over Allen with the grace only an honest-to-God 6'2" natural blonde with great posture and amazing pecs could carry off – a power Big Dick somewhere along the line had finally realized he was entitled to. So now Allen was awake at nights exercising his right hand over this guy who used to be like a total Why Bother?

Allen felt like chopped liver walking down the street with Big Dick. Real old chopped liver. The only people who looked at Allen were very clearly thinking, "Give it up, you geek." Allen feared someone would spit on him for daring to trot along beside Superman as if he thought he'd actually earned it.

And he hadn't. Even though he knew he made Big Dick laugh. Even though the one time that Allen had actually taken at date to a party at the Dicks', Little Dick had made a drunken pass at the guy and ruined everyone's evening. Even though Allen basically (but silently) hated Little Dick, which left Allen in the position not too many friends of lovers-breaking-up were in: He was friends with the *good* one. He wouldn't have to agonize over which side to take or even try to stay friendly with both Dicks. But maybe, since Big Dick was not the type to stay single for more than a week and a half, Allen would be there to help him through his pain and wind up as the new Mrs. Big Dick, and he could carry Big Dick away to an island somewhere and they would both write novels and read comic books and make each other laugh and never be lonely again.

Except that Big Dick was a 6'2" natural blond God and, being a God, he was obligated to fall in love with another God. And Allen, at best, was a sprite.

So Allen did what short guys and plain guys and chubby guys everywhere did when the man they worshipped and wanted to spend the rest of their lives with became available: Allen became Big Dick's Best Friend and Official Matchmaker. As they went to the movies, or out to dinner, Big Dick would smile at only the truly beautiful men while Allen would scream inside, "Me! Me! Choose ME!" hoping that Big Dick would register it telepathically. But Allen would *say,* "Oooooh! Look at that stud over there! He's gorgeous, Dick, and he's cruising you!"

Big Dick would say, "Really?" with the infuriating uncertainty beautiful people have when someone they think is more beautiful than they are is checking them out. And Allen would push Big Dick off toward yet another evening of Godliness and Allenlessness and then go home alone.

When Dick asked Allen why he was always pushing him to have sex with strangers, Allen told Dick he was helping him find his new husband. When Dick asked why Allen wouldn't be his new husband, Allen started to cry and told Big Dick not to tease him. When Dick kissed him, Allen was sure he was going to stop breathing. When Dick told Allen he thought he was falling in love with him, Allen said they better stop kissing and have a talk.

Dick told Allen he thought Allen wasn't interested in him because Allen was always pushing him away, and Allen told Dick he couldn't bear being rejected one more time, and Dick said Allen was the only friend who had stuck by him through his divorce and the only person who really made him laugh and all he could think about was making love to Allen.

When Allen told Dick he was HIV-positive, Dick started to cry. He said it was just his luck and he was probably being punished for leaving Little Dick. Allen said it was okay, they didn't have to do anything, they could just cuddle, but when Big Dick sobbed, "You shouldn't have made me fall in love with you! You shouldn't have done it! I can't handle all this pain!", Allen went home.

Allen never saw Big Dick again.

Estate Sale

by Mark Haile

"That jacket looks perfect on you," he says. The leather slides on silently. The weight is pronounced; the feel, seductive.

Looking through the closet I come across a variety of herringbone tweeds, cashmere, camel hair, banker's gray, navy blue blazers, then on to bomber jackets, fleece gym wear and yet another, more debauched, leather jacket.

In a momentary flash I am reminded of the museum in Berlin which illustrates how the Nazis systematically catalogued the possessions left behind by the concentration camp-bound Jews. I quickly leave the bedroom.

There is crystal enough to cover the breakfast bar, the formal dining table and a small buffet service. A rolling tea cart is crammed with Deco and Streamline bar ware. There is Franciscan tableware to fill several shops.

I surmise the age of the collector by all the memorabilia of female icons planted about the apartment: the late Piaf to early Bette period.

My guide through these remnants of the recently departed's life appears to have been his close friend. Swathed in the leather jacket, I seem to have filled an image reincarnate of the deceased, for now he insists I must take it, continually adjusting the price in a downward spiral as incentive.

Nearly every *tchotchke* I have ever desired or thought worthy of purchase seems present, and I feel safe in assuming that those items that are missing were probably bought by the more astute scavengers of such sales, who know to arrive at the crack of dawn for the most rare of treasures.

This is no haphazard garage sale. There is a meticulous accounting of the stock by my host, with recall of anecdotes regarding the occasions that prompted purchases, original retail prices and current market values. My theory as to the relationship of my guide through this boutique of the dead is thus confirmed: no lover could speak so lovingly of household wares, while simultaneously maintaining his sense of detachment.

My sensibility in regard to the value of such things demands that I take the jacket. He seems relieved. I wonder if his insistence came from a wish to remove from this place the memory this jacket holds – perhaps a reminder of a death that travelled by desire. Or maybe it was just out of want for one less obstacle, in his dual role of salesman and executor, to the goal of selling down to the bare walls.

Once home, the dead man's jacket goes directly to the back of the closet, the section reserved for clothes that I have grown weary of or for other reasons do not wear but cannot bear to part with. It remains unworn; the guilt outweighs the leather.

Coco

by Tracy Cave

Coco the clown was dead. The rumors about his being gay were true. I saw him when he had first been diagnosed with AIDS, after he'd lost fifteen pounds and was suffering from a loss of energy. The fan mail from his afternoon kiddie show, where he hosted cartoons and wished boys and girls happy birthday, had dropped off. I was waiting around the studio for my friend Mitch one day and happened to catch Coco taping his show. A little girl crawled up in his lap, and he lost control of his bowels. Cut. What the hell was going on, the director wanted to know. Didn't he know that children could be traumatized by sitting in clown shit?

Coco was quiet. "AIDS," he said simply, "Goddamn fucking AIDS." The expletives were chilling, coming as they did from a large red smile. Coco pulled off his nose, crumpling it in his hands. "Shit!" said the big red grin.

The station managers had been very nice to Coco. They had given him severance pay, his vacation time, and their wishes for a speedy recovery. It was a very tidy separation. Everyone on the crew had signed the get well card, chosen for the poignancy of the Emmett Kelly face on the front shedding a large, pendulous tear and the simple message inside: "Get Well Soon." Even the homophobic asshole who supervised construction and made off-color jokes about Coco behind his back signed the card. All that was missing was an engraved gold watch, and Coco could have pretended that he was taking an early retirement.

Only none of us would have believed that. He was, after all, a shadow of his former self. Meanwhile, the station was doing everything it could to mollify the parents of the little girl who had sat in Coco's lap. "Must have gotten hold of a nasty bug," the P.R. lady had reassured the girl's father, "and please, won't you and your family enjoy a day at Disneyland on us?" And things like, "Our sponsors would like you to accept a year's supply of apple/blueberry/banana instant drink mix, fortified with seven essential vitamins and minerals." The P.R. lady laid it on thick; she was a walking commercial, for Christ's sake.

If I had been the kid's father, I wouldn't have believed that line of bull, not for a minute. I'd figure there was something fishy going on. I'd want to know if my kid was just shit on, or was she shit on by someone with AIDS – now there's a suit for you. Threaten to break it to the press and settle for a tidy sum outside of court. The people who make the instant apple/blueberry crap have money, which is amazing enough considering what the stuff tastes like. But I guess the station hit it lucky: an especially dim family of heteros who hadn't been to Disneyland in quite a while.

Forget about them, let's get back to Coco, the late, great clown. Coco didn't hang on for a long time after his ignominious departure from the kiddie show. he was, to put it bluntly, one gloomy clown. And who could blame him? The poor guy could barely get off the toilet seat. Soon, he had to be hospitalized with dehydration, and he never went back home except for a few days once or twice. After his death, I helped pack up his things. Would you believe the guy owned nine pairs of pajama bottoms?

You'd think that, my having helped him on the toilet and packing up his pj's, I had been his best friend, but in fact, I hardly knew the guy. In truth my best friend Mitch was the one who knew Coco. Yes, had even known him in the carnal sense, but that was back in college. Mitch had brought out Coco, who was then called Brad or Bruce or something like that (no, it couldn't have been Bruce; I'd have remembered that.) Now Mitch says that Brad/Coco brought him out, but from the way he says it and the sort of hazy way he remembers it, I can tell it was the other way around. Well, I mean, that's how well I know Mitch. Anyway, so Mitch, you know, is the cute fortyish weather forecaster on Channel 9 with the fake grey streaks at his temples. Yes, you know him. Didn't you know he was gay? Well, I think it's so obvious. Now, Mitch and Coco had been friends at college, but they didn't meet up again until about two years before Coco's death.

He had been an actor on the legitimate stage – mostly off-Broadway, mostly gay avant-garde theater – well, just try making a living at that. So, a friend of a friend got him this job out here as a clown on a kiddie show. Hey, what are you going to do? He needed a job, with real benefits. Lucky he had the hospitalization. I mean, can you imagine if he had still been working at his art? Who'd have changed his shit-filled pajamas then? But I digress. So, one day after he had just started working as a clown, Coco came stomping off the set (probably a kid had just bitten him) and literally ran smack into Mitch, who looks, except for the grey temples, just as he did in college. Coco grabbed him and planted a big old sweaty clown kiss right on Mitch's cheek. Not recognizing Coco, Mitch though he was being raped by a psychotic circus clown. When they got it all straightened out, it was too late for Mitch to redo his makeup, so he had to go on and talk about hurricanes with clown lips smeared down his cheek and the anchorman making all these hetero innuendos about Mitch's prowess with the ladies. Geez! Mitch is about as smooth with the ladies as Coco was with the kids.

I'm not saying Coco wasn't a good clown. Like any good actor, he threw himself into the role, reading about the lives of famous clowns and studying their history way back to the commedia dell'arte. I think he even went away to a summer training thing for clowns. But the fact of the matter is, he didn't care a whole lot for the kids. If you looked closely, you could see that in his performance, though I'd never have told him that. I didn't even meet him until after he'd gotten sick. And then for some reason, he and I hit it off. I could tell that Mitch wasn't going to be much help. He means well and promises the world, but if I were in Coco's shoes, I wouldn't want to depend on Mitch as my basis for support. He's a flake, pure and simple. In all the years I've known him, he has never shown up to dinner on time. Sometimes he forgets entirely. It's just about all he can do to keep his grey hair corralled at his temples.

So the beginning of the end was that Mitch made all these promises (which I am sure he fully intended to keep), and I was the one who ended up taking on the care and feeding of Coco the clown. I guess I'm beginning to sound like a martyr, but actually, it wasn't so bad. Coco lives, or rather lived, near me, so I could just pop over a few times a day and wash up the pj's and the dishes. He slept a lot, but when he was awake, we'd talk a little about his life in New York and about his college days with Mitch. He told me he used to call Mitch a BDWB (Big Dick Without Brains), and sometimes, when he was tired and depressed, he'd talk about what he would have done if he hadn't gotten AIDS. Can you believe he wanted to go back to the theater? He wanted to save enough money from being Coco the clown to go back to New York and try it again. I've really got to hand it to him on that; I sold out years ago. I was either going to play violin in a major metropolitan orchestra or get my Ph.D. in geology and teach at some cushy university. When neither of these happened, I settled for teaching geology part-time at the community colleges. I teach geo labs one morning and three afternoons a week, resting my hand on the well-muscled jocks as I explain the difference between igneous and sedimentary rocks. They seldom get it, but I offer tons of extra help and pass them anyway. The track coach is a friend of Bertha's, if you catch my drift, and always sends me a choice group of students, and for that, I pass them all. Not a bad system, but it's not exactly the fulfillment of all my dreams.

I guess we all die with some of our dreams unfulfilled. Coco did. He died two months ago. Now that I think of it, his real name was Brian and he changed it to Brad, or it was Brad and he changed it to Brian. I don't think either one is much of a stage name, but then I called him Coco right up until the end. The last time I saw him, he was in a coma with tubes running from all over his body. In a way, I knew it was the last time I'd see him, and I'd wished there were some way I could have said good-bye to him, but he was already out of it. I wasn't surprised the next day when Mitch called and told me that Coco had died during the night. The body was to be cremated and shipped back East to some brothers who never visited him when he was sick. Mitch said he would make the arrangements for a memorial service.

Mitch, as usual, flaked out, and I ended up arranging the service. We had it at a Unitarian church. I think Coco was agnostic. Mitch and I managed to get together about forty gay friends for the service, so there were those friends and a handful of people from the station. The station sent a large wreath with a clown face in the center, and some executive from the station, who had probably never met Coco, stood up and spoke in a grave voice about how much joy Brian or Brad had given to all the children. I nearly puked. Everyone else was obviously moved, though, so I refrained. Mitch gave the main eulogy and talked about their college days and told the story of how he had to do the weather one day with a big red clown kiss on his cheek. I doubt that Coco would have chosen to be remembered like this. But it was the best we all could do.

I remember once when he wasn't in much pain and was talking about what he'd do if they found a cure for AIDS tomorrow, I asked him how he could stand to be a TV clown after having been a real actor in New York. He just shrugged and said, "You do what you have to do."

I think about that now. When Coco was in the hospital, I finally got up the nerve to have the test. You know, *the test.* The results weren't surprising, but no matter how prepared you think you are, you aren't prepared to hear that there's a time bomb in your body that could go off any day. It could explode clown shit everywhere.

How Not to Get Attached to a Fish

by David Vernon

Someone gives you a live fish. Work hard to recognize that this was meant as a kind gesture. Don't say, "No, thanks, I'm not the fish sort of person." Don't tell this friend that you can barely remember to feed yourself these days. Accept the small tank and the fish and say, "Thank you."

Put the tank on a nightstand away from the bed, moving a stack of Bruce's drawing pads that you should have packed away by now.

Try not to gaze at the fish for too long, for although you know the fish is blue, the closer you study it gliding about the tank the more you notice the greens and yellows and subtle shadings of tangerine.

Casually crumble a few saltines into the tank while you attempt, once again, to read chapter two of *The Unbearable Lightness of Being,* hoping this time you might see the words as parts of a sentence with meaning and not just as scratches of ink on a piece of paper.

Try not to get too alarmed the next morning when you notice that the fish hasn't eaten the soggy wad of cracker resting on the bottom of his tank. Be casual. Grab some clothes you've been meaning to drop off at the AIDS thrift shop and make going to the pet store just another errand.

Act detached, even impatient as you show the clerk the fish and ask her what it eats and what kind of fish it is. Restrain yourself from taking out a pen and notepad when she tells you the exotic name, a Beta, for the type of fish you now own. Be suitably disgusted when she hands you a Styrofoam cup filled with tiny live worms. As you are getting change back from your dollar, ask the clerk what other fish are compatible with yours. And when she tells you that it is the only kind of fish that absolutely must live alone, try not to ache at the realization that you and this fish might have something in common after all.

When friends ask you the fish's name reply quickly, "No name; it's just a stupid fish." Throw an annoyed stare at the person who says, "Oh, you're just trying not to get attached."

Curse the fish as you gouge through the worm pulp with a plastic fork, separating a live worm from the mass of dead ones and toss it into the tank to be devoured by your fish. Wonder out loud why this friend of yours couldn't have given you sea monkeys or an ant farm.

Reassure yourself that it is "Jeopardy" and the dashing Alex Trebek and not your fish that is making you hurry home from work.

Justify naming him Scotty by telling yourself that by naming him after a character from "Star Trek," your least favorite show, you will have no trouble giving him away when you have the chance.

Pretend not to notice that Scotty propels his fins madly and seems genuinely glad to see you when you come home from work. And on his second cup of worms don't acknowledge a tinge of warmth as you dangle a worm just beneath the surface of the tank and Scotty swims to the top and eats it off your fork.

Worry a bit when a friend who is checking in on you notes, "You can really tell that that fish loves you."

Allow yourself to be concerned when you catch yourself coming home from work and telling Scotty about your day. Say to the fish, "I do not care about you. I refuse to care about anyone or anything ever again." Convince yourself that you are just talking out loud as you tell Scotty about Bruce; about your six years together; about his handsome dark looks and light olive complexion. About the vacation the two of you took in Spain. About how you feel adrift and out to sea on the king-size bed without him. Know that it's time to turn off the light and sleep when you hear yourself whispering to Scotty, "Bruce would have loved you."

Don't be annoyed when your mother calls and asks you about your fish. Don't point out that in all your years together and throughout his illness that she never once asked about Bruce.

Refrain from telling anyone at work how you really spent your Sunday, gazing into this fish tank, noticing how the fish uses his pelvic fins almost like landing gear to anchor himself. Don't tell them that you forgot about time as you watched Scotty hover and swim. Don't mention how you wondered if Scotty stares at you and sees you trapped in your own aquarium, populated with dying plants and a cardboard backdrop. Control yourself, as your co-workers discuss gallery openings and "60 Minutes," from telling them what you learned about tranquility and acceptance in one day from a fish.

Be calm when you return home from work, finding the cleaning woman your mother hired vacuuming the carpet and you see an empty tank laying by your bed. Don't show any emotion as the cleaning lady, using a combination of fractured English and pantomime explains to you how she found the fish floating belly-up. "Is gone," she tells you, "I flush down toilet."

When you find yourself depressed, blame it on other things: the war, another bad haircut. Listen and even agree with the friend who says to you, "Life goes in cycles. There is peace in accepting that."

When the man at work who always wears gray suits, even on t-shirt day, remarks that you look distant, don't tell him that you are trying to remember exactly where water flushed down the toilet goes. To an ocean, perhaps? Don't tell this person that you are needing to find a place to picture Scotty, someplace like a deep, warm Mediterranean sea filled with color and wonder and cycles.

See this co-worker standing next to you, puzzled by your silence. You want to control and restrain, hold back and pull in. Then a tiny dam breaks. A light turns on. A window opens. A taut muscle relaxes. You find that you are weary from control and denial. You start to cry, not even worrying about what anyone around you will think. You even get your co-worker's sleeve damp before he flees the scene. Pretty soon you've cleared out the entire hallway. You sit on the carpet and realize that you regret all the missed opportunities of saying good-bye. Good-bye to Eric, whom you captured and tied up during your high school Halloween party. Two years older than you, he was the first boy you ever wanted. You finally had him alone, his arms and legs bound together. His glare told you that you could do anything to him. You pushed the first bottle of poppers you owned under his nose, stroked his hard nipples, then ran away, leaving him tied up because you didn't know what to do next. You hear that he's gone now. Good-bye to Andra who has it and is still missing. Good-bye to Rodney who died overseas. Good-bye to Ricardo who died when you were away at school. Good-bye to William, who killed himself when he found out, standing you up for lunch at Trumps. Good-bye to Lucille who said that he got it from sharing needles with Nancy Reagan. Good-bye to Scotty, flushed down the toilet.

Ever since Bruce's family had his body cremated, his ashes disposed of against your wishes, you've needed to picture Bruce squatting on a stretch of plain like the one you hiked up to outside of Barcelona. It was flat like the way they once believed the whole world to be and quiet like the day after time. You close your eyes and you see Bruce on this plain. Bruce slightly unshaven. Bruce stretching. Making a connection. You understanding finally the concept of cycles. And him just sitting there looking gorgeous.

Contributors

Luis Alfaro is a performance artist who was born and raised in the Pico-Union district of downtown Los Angeles. He is the recipient of a Brody Arts Fellowship, and grants from the California Arts Council and Los Angeles Department of Cultural Affairs. Luis wrote and performed "Downtown" through workshops at the Mark Taper Forum, Sushi Gallery and Footworks; the piece premiered at Highways Performance Space. Luis is currently in the Mentor Playwrights Program at the Mark Taper Forum. He is the manager of The Gathering Place, a drop-in center for people with HIV, ARC and AIDS in South Central Los Angeles.

Paul Attinello: I am a musician, writer, and voracious reader, born in 1956. After brief experiences of eastern cities, I made San Francisco my home in 1979; I went into exile in Los Angeles in 1984 to study musicology at UCLA. My poems and short fiction date from 1989; I am published in *West Coast Plays* as co-author of San Francisco's long-running *The AIDS Show*, and in the Los Angeles Festival anthology *Harbinger*. As a gay man with ARC, I've been intimately involved with the loneliness and sorrow of the epidemic, which seem to me more terrible than illness and death.

Tracy Cave has been writing in Terry Wolverton's writing classes ever since he saw a 1988 ad in a local gay rag for her HIV+ writer's group. Testing positive in 1986 and becoming a PWA in 1990, he has found writing about AIDS to be an apt way of dealing with his feelings and channeling those feelings into creativity. Currently, this Aquarian is living in North Hollywood with his computer, boa constrictor and rat. He writes short fiction that sometimes deals with AIDS and sometimes not. He teaches composition classes at local community colleges and also works as a sign language interpreter.

Gil Cuadros is a native Angeleno, PWARC and HIV educator. "At the end of 1987, AIDS totally devastated my life; my lover died suddenly, I was diagnosed with the fatal disease and all my 25-year-old aspirations were killed. Out of this hell I found two things: I wanted to write, and I was a survivor. My new life is built on this simple but strong foundation."

Terri de la Peña: The "Frankie" in my life died in 1986, one month before my father. We were childhood friends and I suspected his gayness long before recognizing my lesbian self. After my coming out, we spoke often about the differences between Chicano gays and Chicano lesbians, the varying options and limitations imposed by our culture. We did not always agree, *pero reímos mucho.* I wish he were here to share more talk, to read my stories, to keep making me laugh. He left much too soon, and I like to think I'm living for us both.

Paul Decker dropped out of show business after spending too many years of his life as NBC's Director of Casting, where he supervised the casting of various soap operas and a host of TV movies about people shooting other people in the head. He is now better known as Alice in Rubberland, in which guise he happily designs and sells rubber stamps. Thanks to Terry Wolverton, without whom this story would never have been started. Or finished.

Ayofemi Folayan is an activist concerned with saving the planet and creating a world of peace and harmony; she pursues the end of all forms of violence and oppression through her creative energy as a writer. She describes writing as the umbilical cord from the universe which nurtures her spirit. Her work has been anthologized in *In A Different Light: An Anthology of Lesbian Writers, Spring Street* and *Lesbians at Midlife: The Creative Transition.* Her columns, essays, book reviews and short fiction have appeared in *Gay Community News, Matrix, BLK, off our backs, Sojourner, Vanguard* and the *Advocate.* Ayofemi writes to alleviate her frustration at the deaths from AIDS and breast cancer that have taken away so many of her friends. She is currently working on a new performance piece, "The Talking Drum," and finishing her novel, *Onyx.*

Eric Gutierrez is a writer and performer who started life next door to General Motors in the San Fernando Valley. He used to be a nice boy from the suburbs but since 1987 has been acting up, fighting back and trying to stop AIDS as a member of ACT UP/LA. "The Go-Go Prince" was presented as a work-in-progress at Highways Performance Space, and premiered at Los Angeles Contemporary Exhibitions (LACE) in May 1991.

Mark Haile is an African-born American of African descent. He is a journalist, poet, songwriter and editor, serving on the staff of *BLK* and *Kuumba.* He is also a coordinator for the literary circle of VIVA. Among the literary events he has organized, Mark curated a reading for A Day Without Art as part of an ongoing effort to support Organization SIDA Tijuana in Baja California, Mexico and the Minority AIDS Project in Los Angeles. He lives in Chinatown Heights overlooking downtown L.A.

Bia Lowe: I can't say what the "metaphor" of AIDS is. I do know it represents a monumental challenge: To live fully in spite of it. To speak powerfully despite indifference to it. To teach what we know about living despite contempt for who we are. To write, as Annie Dillard put it, as if our lives depended on it. My work has appeared in *Caliban, The Beloit Poetry Journal, The Western Humanities Review* and *The California Quarterly*, among other places.

Keith Antar Mason: First off, I am a black working class straight poet… who has friends who are dying alone and ashamed in the Afrikan-American community. I do not understand that. We who came to America in bondage together. Must surely know the value of community. I must struggle against Black Male Silence: the number one killer of black males. I will not tolerate oppression of any kind against my people. I must speak out against homophobia and black male bashing. Peace to the people so the people can have some. Peace. We must learn to love ourselves.

Rondo Mieczkowski: Other excerpts from "The AIDS Dance" appear in *Poetry/L.A.* and *Diseased Pariah News.* My latest poetry chapbook is *Spring & Two Chickens.* I curate the Gay Writers Series at A Different Light Bookstore in L.A. The list of my AIDS dead include Allan, Andrew, Antonio, Billy, Buddy, Bruce, Carl, Carlos, Chuck, Denis, Dennis, Don, Don, Ernesto, Gennaro, Ian, Jean, Jean-Louis, Jerry, Jim, John, Merwyn, Mikel, Neal, Paul, Preston, Richard, Rob, Roger, Ron, Ronnie, Sam, Steven, Steven, Tiffany, Tracey, Vince, Waylon and names I can't remember and names I never knew. All murdered by a neglectful American society.

Tim Miller: I am a performance artist, teacher and cultural organizer. I do my performances and workshops all over this country. I also run around like a nut at Highways Performance Space which I founded with Linda Burnham in 1989. I offer this piece in the spirit of let's get down to it, Oh Dudes and Dudettes, the big job of knowing ourselves, healing society, confronting fear and ACTING UP!

Paul Monette is the author of four books about AIDS: the novels *Halfway Home* and *Afterlife; Borrowed Time: An AIDS Memoir;* and a book of poems, *Love Alone: 18 Elegies for Rog.* He has been fighting this war for so long that he doesn't remember the time before the nightmare anymore, but he's written eleven other books. If only books saved lives. He is currently at work on an autobiography, *Becoming a Man.*

David E. Moores was born October 17, 1948 in a small town in Minnesota. He graduated from St. Cloud University and taught junior high school, before moving to California in 1974. There he worked in the furniture and retail industries, and finally in the training department of Great Western Bank. Following a three-year illness, David died of complications of AIDS. He not only had a great love for God's creation, but had a deep faith. David died peacefully knowing that he was passing into the everlasting arms of Jesus.

Robin Podolsky is a writer of fiction, essays, poetry and drama. Her work has appeared in *In a Different Light,* an anthology of lesbian writing (Clothespin Fever Press), and will be forthcoming in *Indivisible* (New American Library.) Her work-in-progress, *Roughing It Out,* has been awarded a Special Citation by the PEN Center. She is the editor of *Caregiver,* a publication of the AIDS Healthcare Foundation. "AIDS work has reminded me that it's not naive to care intensely about people, ideas or reshaping the world. And that, under the gun, lesbian and gay people can come through."

Aleida Rodríguez co-founded, co-edited, and co-published the first lesbian-run literary magazine and press in Los Angeles, *rara avis* /Books of a Feather, 1978-84. Her writing is included in anthologies nationwide. She feels that too often what gets written about AIDS are memoirs and eulogies, not complex depictions of *living* with the nuances, alert to the epiphanies. "The Surreal Answer the World Hands You" is a portrait of one such moment. Aleida teaches writing in the AIDS unit of the Chino women's prison.

Crespin Rosas: Until I began reading gay and lesbian literature I thought I had no role models. I grew up reading Whitman and Oscar Wilde and grew into a realization of myself. Through books I've learned from Blacks, Jews, the women's movement... and realized progress can be made. I've known no world without AIDS and truly believe we will overcome this disease which has taken far too many. We are writing gay and lesbian history.

Doug Sadownick: I write because, with AIDS having claimed so many of my people, it is one way I give testimony to the women and men who stand up bravely to the assault on our bodies, souls and cultures this holocaust represents. Sometimes fiction or performance art seems appropriate; other times I write for the *L.A. Weekly, L.A. Times,* and the *Advocate.* I grew up in the Bronx, got a B.A. at Columbia, an M.A. at NYU, taught English at universities in New York and Los Angeles. Now I'm writing a novel about the way AIDS rattles the psychological cages of a lower-middle-class Jewish family.

Susan Silton is a designer and visual artist with roots in writing. "First my cousin died of AIDS in the early 80's, when people couldn't even remember the acronym much less what it stood for.We were the only queers in the family, so there was an undeniable bond, but my fear ran rampant through the course of his illness. Then, years later, I fell for a woman who told me she had AIDS on our second date. I am forever grateful to that relationship for what it taught me about love & friendship, the body's fragility and the soul's resiliency."

David Vernon lives in Los Angeles. His work can be seen in *Indivisible,* an upcoming anthology from New American Library. "An assignment in a recent writing workshop proposed: 'Write about someone who loses something and gains something else.' It occurred to me that this was the theme of much of my recent writing. Almost a decade of the AIDS crisis has for me been like surviving a nightmarish shipwreck. Standing on the beach, clothes in tatters, debris washing ashore, you ask yourself, how did this happen, why am I here and what now?

Alan Zimmerman was born in 1943 in Petaluma, California. After four years in the Air Force, he studied art at the College of Marin and the California College of Arts & Crafts. While continuing to produce art, he worked as an airbrush artist and doing construction and renovation work. His exhibitions included those at Permanent Contemporary Gallery, Thinking Eye Gallery, La Luz de Jesus, and Ankrum Gallery. He also created altars for the Healing Light Center in Glendale, California. He died on August 24, 1990 of complications related to AIDS.

Terry Wolverton (Editor): In 1988 I began teaching a creative writing workshop for people with HIV; I am moved and inspired by the clarity and honesty in the work of these men. The bullshit is largely stripped away, because there's no more time for it. My own fiction, poetry, drama and art criticism have appeared in numerous periodicals and anthologies. I recently served as poetry editor for *Harbinger: poetry and fiction by Los Angeles writers* and as co-editor of *Indivisible: short fiction by west coast lesbians and gays.* I am hard at work on my first novel, *The Labrys Reunion.*